Full-Field Digital Mammography

CASE-BASED APPROACH

Full-Field Digital Mammography

CASE-BASED APPROACH

Anurag Jain MD, FRCR

Senior Consultant and Head
Department of Radiology
Action Cancer Hospital, Delhi

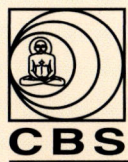

CBS

CBS Publishers & Distributors Pvt Ltd

New Delhi • Bengaluru • Chennai • Kochi • Kolkata • Mumbai
Bhopal • Bhubaneswar • Hyderabad • Jharkhand • Nagpur • Patna
• Pune • Uttarakhand • Dhaka (Bangladesh)

Full-Field Digital Mammography
CASE-BASED APPROACH

ISBN: 978-93-89396-27-0

Copyright © Author and Publisher

First Edition: 2020

Published by Satish Kumar Jain and produced by Varun Jain for

CBS Publishers & Distributors Pvt Ltd

4819/XI Prahlad Street, 24 Ansari Road, Daryaganj, New Delhi 110 002, India.
Ph: 23289259, 23266861, 23266867   Website: www.cbspd.com
Fax: 011-23243014   e-mail: delhi@cbspd.com; cbspubs@airtelmail.in.

Corporate Office: 204 FIE, Industrial Area, Patparganj, Delhi 110 092
Ph: 4934 4934   Fax: 4934 4935   e-mail: publishing@cbspd.com; publicity@cbspd.com

Branches

• **Bengaluru:** Seema House 2975, 17th Cross, K.R. Road,
  Banasankari 2nd Stage, Bengaluru 560 070, Karnataka
  Ph: +91-80-26771678/79   Fax: +91-80-26771680   e-mail: bangalore@cbspd.com
• **Chennai:** 7, Subbaraya Street, Shenoy Nagar, Chennai 600 030, Tamil Nadu
  Ph: +91-44-26680620, 26681266   Fax: +91-44-42032115   e-mail: chennai@cbspd.com
• **Kochi:** 42/1325, 1326, Power House Road, Opp KSEB Power House,
  Ernakulam 682 018, Kochi, Kerala
  Ph: +91-484-4059061-65   Fax: +91-484-4059065   e-mail: kochi@cbspd.com
• **Kolkata:** 6/B, Ground Floor, Rameswar Shaw Road, Kolkata-700 014, West Bengal
  Ph: +91-33-22891126, 22891127, 22891128   e-mail: kolkata@cbspd.com
• **Mumbai:** 83-C, Dr E Moses Road, Worli, Mumbai-400018, Maharashtra
  Ph: +91-22-24902340/41   Fax: +91-22-24902342   e-mail: mumbai@cbspd.com

Representatives

• **Bhopal**	0-8319310552	• **Bhubaneswar**	0-9911037372	• **Hyderabad**	0-9885175004
• **Jharkhand**	0-9811541605	• **Nagpur**	0-9421945513	• **Patna**	0-9334159340
• **Pune**	0-9623451994	• **Uttarakhand**	0-9716462459	• **Dhaka (Bangladesh)**	01912-003485

Printed at: Magic International Pvt. Ltd., Greater Noida, UP, India

This book gives a compilation of mammography appearances in diverse breast abnormalities with emphasis on the varied presentations of breast cancer. The collection includes cases of early breast cancers which are clinically occult and picked up on screening mammography. Key points are included in all cases to emphasize various practical aspects in the approach to interpretation and work-up of breast abnormalities on mammography. Nearly all included cases are proved on histopathology and their pathology appearances are presented along side.

Anurag Jain

Acknowledgment

I would like to thank Mr. SK Jain, Chairman and Managing Director, CBS Publishers & Distributors Pvt. Ltd. for his support in bringing out this high resolution mammography Atlas of Full-Field Digital Mammography giving a case-based approach. All the cases were done on 'Fuji Amulet' mammography machine at Action Cancer Hospital and I thank the Fuji India team for their excellent application support with special mention of Ms Swati Sharma.

CREDITS

Action Cancer Hospital

Dr Asha Agarwal
Medical Superintendent

Dr Naveen Agarwal, MD
Senior Consultant and Head,
Department of Pathology

Dr Sheena Khetarpal, MD
Consultant, Department of Pathology

Ms Jyotsana Tanwar
Mammography Technologist

My Strength
Vandana (my wife)
Avnika and Mihika (my daughters)

My Inspiration

Smt Pushpa Jain (my mother)
Shri SCK Jain (my father)

Contents

Breast cancer is the commonest cancer in females worldwide, representing a quarter of all cancers. In India also, breast cancer is the number one cancer in women with an estimated age adjusted rate of 25.8 per 100,000 women and mortality of 12.7 per 100,000 women according to a recent publication by S Malvia, et al (Asia-Pacific Journal of Clinical Oncology 2017; 13: 289–295). The age-adjusted incidence of breast carcinoma is highest in the big cities of India, being 41 per 100,000 women for Delhi, followed by Chennai (37.9), **Bengaluru** (34.4) and Thiruvananthapuram (33.7).

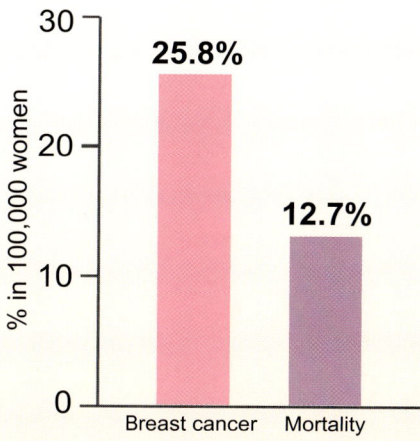

Although the incidence of breast cancer is lower in rural areas, the mortality/incidence ratio is as high as 66.3%, compared to 8% in Delhi. In rural areas, cancer patients are diagnosed at late or advanced stages of disease with a higher proportion of them having widespread metastasis.

An ICMR survey in the metropolitan cities has shown that the incidence of breast cancer almost doubled in the period between 1982 and 2005. The average age at diagnosis of breast cancer in Indian women is nearly 10 years lower as compared to western women. Further worrying is the fact that breast cancer is generally more aggressive in behavior in younger patients. Studies suggest that the disease peaks at 40–50 years in Indian women. Unfortunately, majority of Indian patients present at locally advanced or metastatic stages at the time of diagnosis.

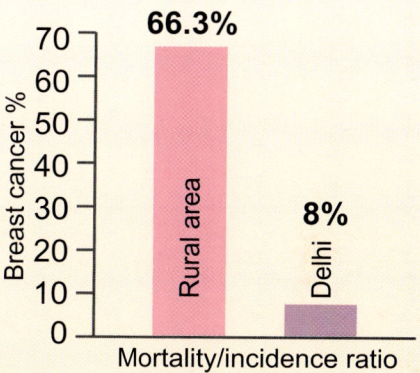

As per Globocon, breast cancer is the second most common cause of cancer mortality after lung cancer. The incidence of breast cancer rises steadily with age in premenopausal state, there being a decline in the rate of rise in incidence after menopause. Obesity and increased lifetime exposure to estrogens and progesterone as seen in women with early age at menarche (<12 years), late

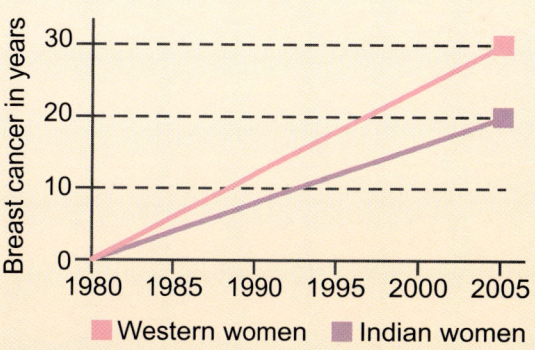

menopause (>55 years) and low parity are known risk factors for breast cancer. Exposure to environmental toxins, such as lipophilic polycyclic aromatic hydrocarbons, is also considered a risk factor. In about 5% of breast cancer cases, there is a strong familial risk mediated by mutations in BRCA1 and BRCA2 genes inherited from parents. These mutations are also noted in about 2.8% of early-onset breast cancer patients in the India. Physical activity and longer duration of breastfeeding are protective against breast cancer.

Late presentation due to various factors including lack of awareness, poor educational and socio-economic status, lower concern towards the health and wellness of women in many sections of Indian society lead to higher mortality in Indian breast cancer patients. Factors, such as inequities in the health infrastructure availability, lack of organized breast cancer screening programs and paucity of diagnostic tools and equipment also contribute to late detection and higher mortality.

A multipronged approach to breast cancer is needed with emphasis on preventive measures, awareness and screening programs. Availability of diagnostic and treatment facilities is also imperative for reducing the incidence as well as mortality related to breast cancer in Indian women.

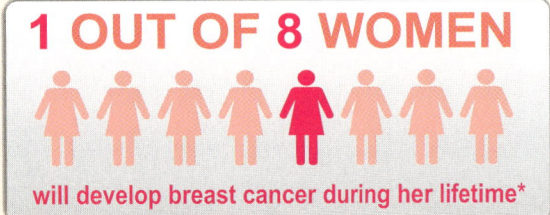

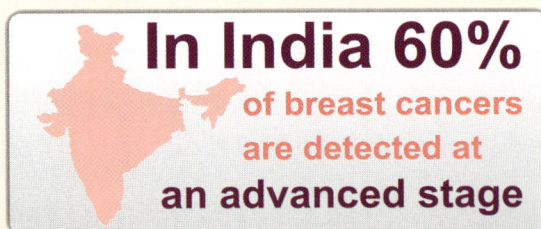

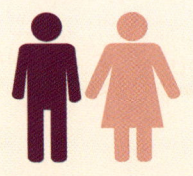

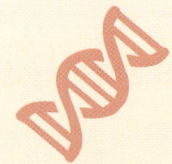

⚠ BEING A WOMAN

Breast cancer is **100x** more common among women

⚠ AGING

2 out of 3 invasive breast cancers are found in women age 55 or older

⚠ GENETICS

5-10% of breast cancer cases are hereditary

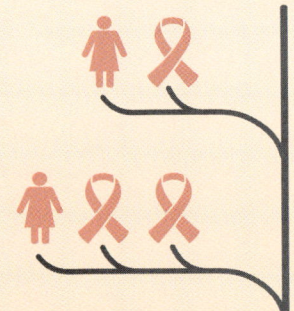

⚠ FAMILY HISTORY

Having one first-degree relative with breast cancer approximately **doubles a woman's risk**

Having two first-degree relatives increases her risk about **3-fold**

⚠ PERSONAL HISTORY

A woman with cancer in one breast has a **3- to 4-fold increased risk** of developing new breast caner

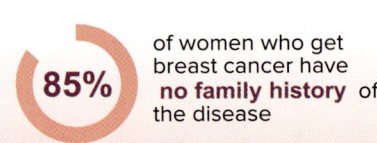

85% of women who get breast cancer have **no family history** of the disease

CASE STUDIES

MLO: Mediolateral oblique view   HPE: Histopathological examination
CC: Craniocaudal view   FNAC: Fine needle aspiration cytology

Normal appearance: ACR Type A density

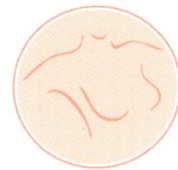

Mammography

ACR Type A density: Both breasts are predominantly fatty with fibroglandular parenchyma comprising <25% of breast.

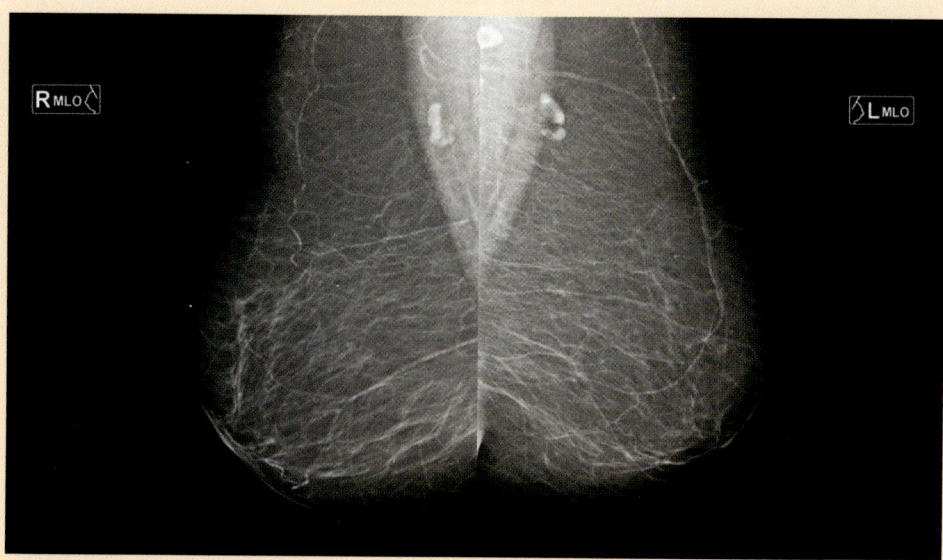

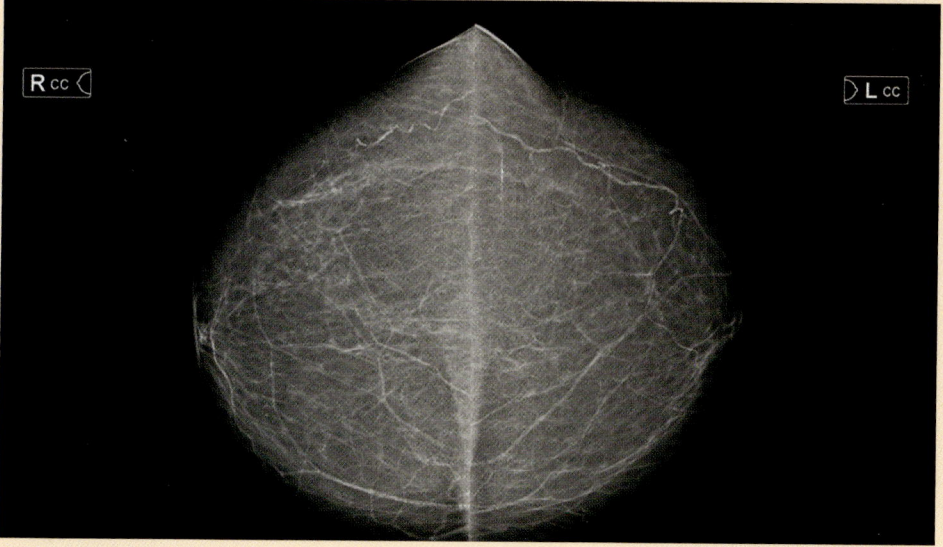

Key Points

Breasts are predominantly low attenuating due to sparse glandular component. Mammography is most sensitive in detecting abnormalities in predominantly fatty breasts as the soft tissue lesions and microcalcifications stand out in the background of low attenuating breasts. Small volume axillary nodes with fatty hilum are not abnormal.

Normal appearance: ACR Type B density

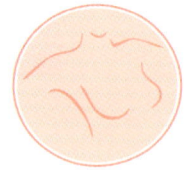

Mammography

ACR Type B density: Scattered fibroglandular parenchyma comprising 25–50% of breast.

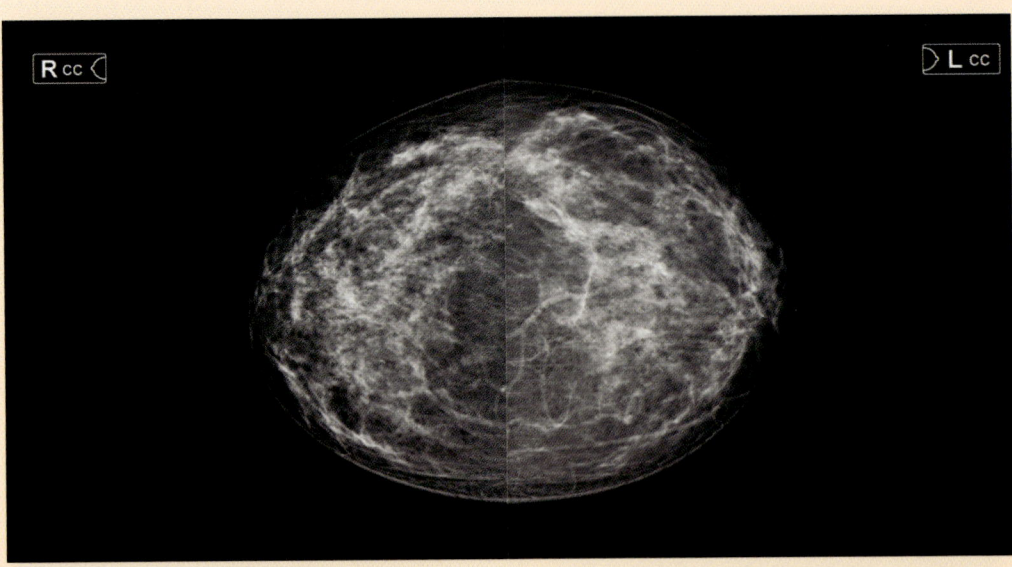

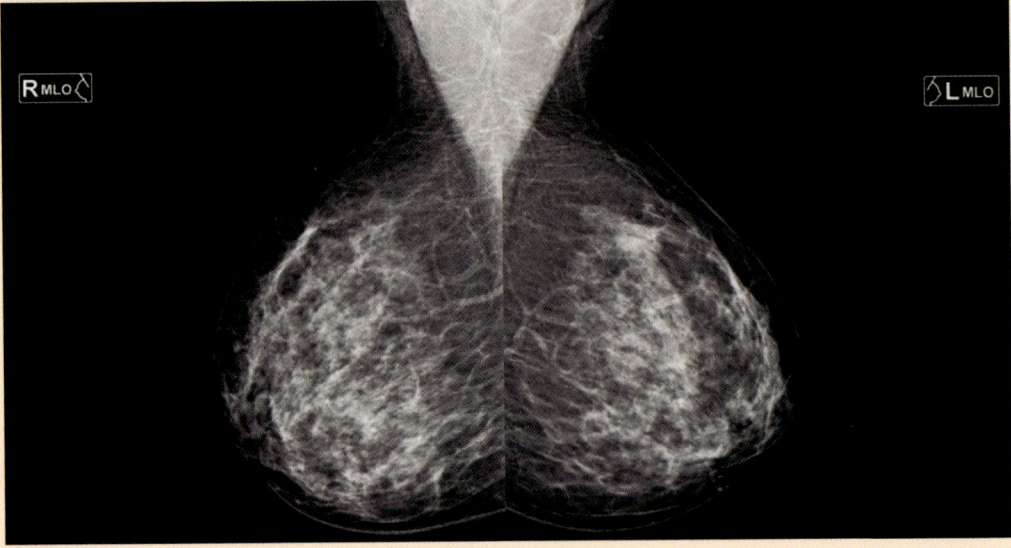

Key Points

Relatively easier to evaluate for abnormalities as compared to Type C/D breast compositions. Look for focal asymmetry, focal soft tissue lesions, architectural distortion or localized microcalcifications.

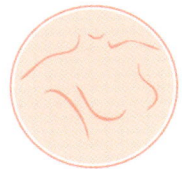

Normal appearance: ACR Type C density

Mammography

ACR Type C density: Heterogeneous firboglandular parenchyma comprising 50–75% of breast.

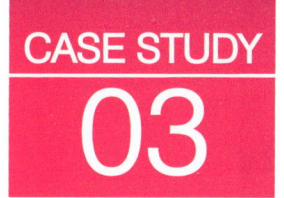

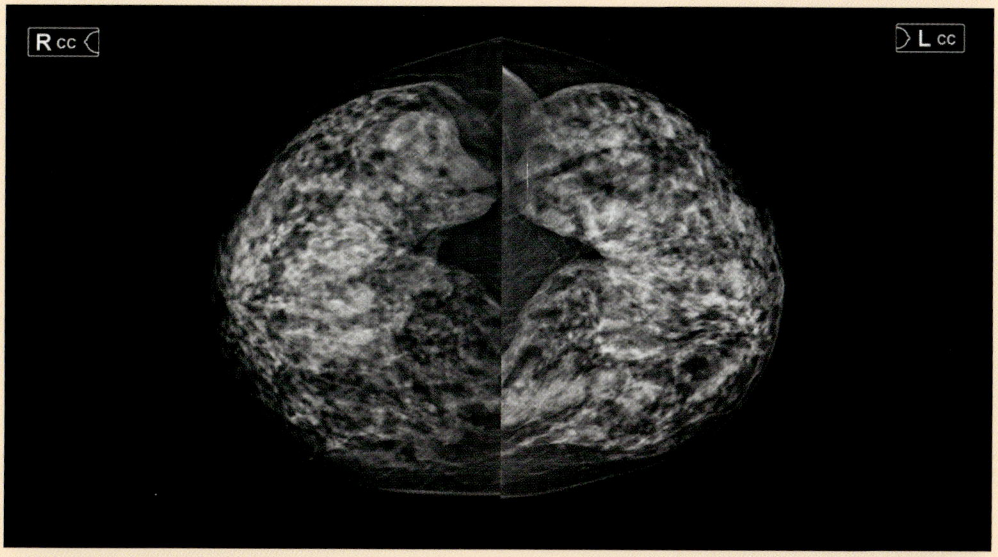

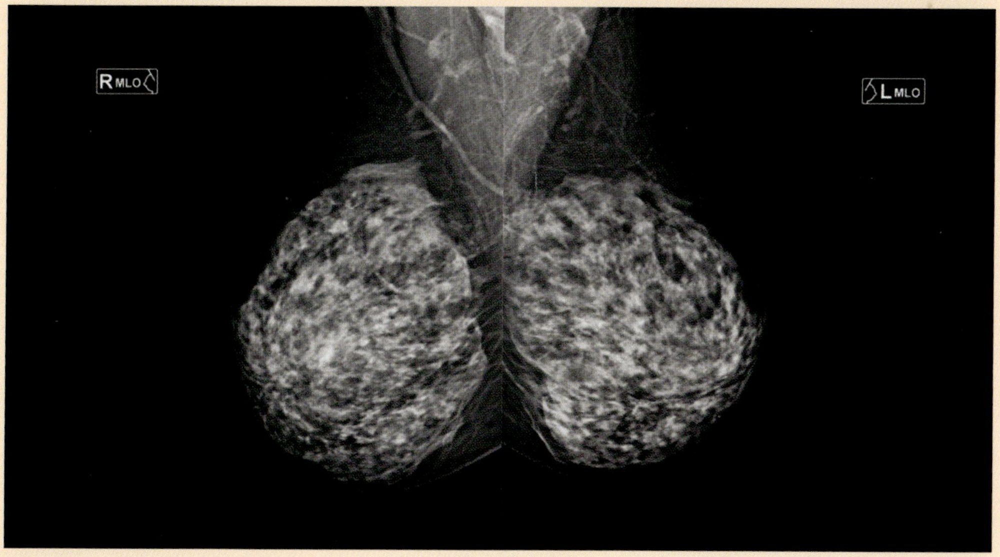

Key Points

It is difficult to evaluate for focal abnormalities due to heterogeneously dense breast attenuation. Meticulous quadrant wise evaluation should be done for focal abnormalities. Extra views, like spot rolled/spot compression/magnification views, may need to be taken for confirmation of abnormalities.

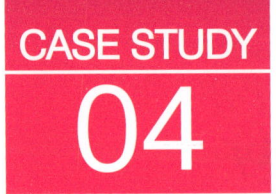

Normal appearance: ACR Type D density

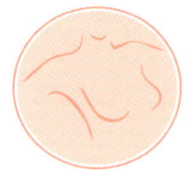

Mammography

ACR Type D density: Extremely dense breast parenchyma comprising >75% breast.

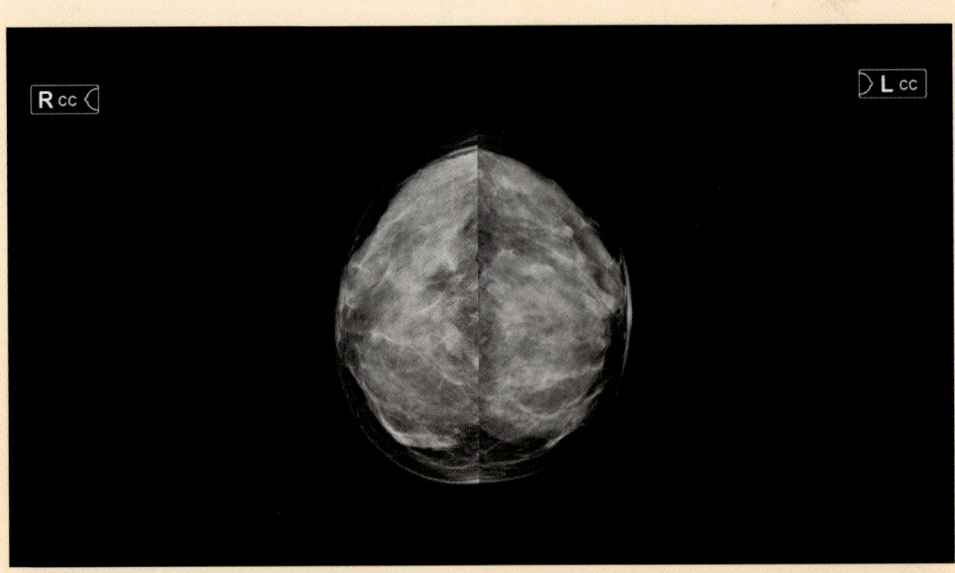

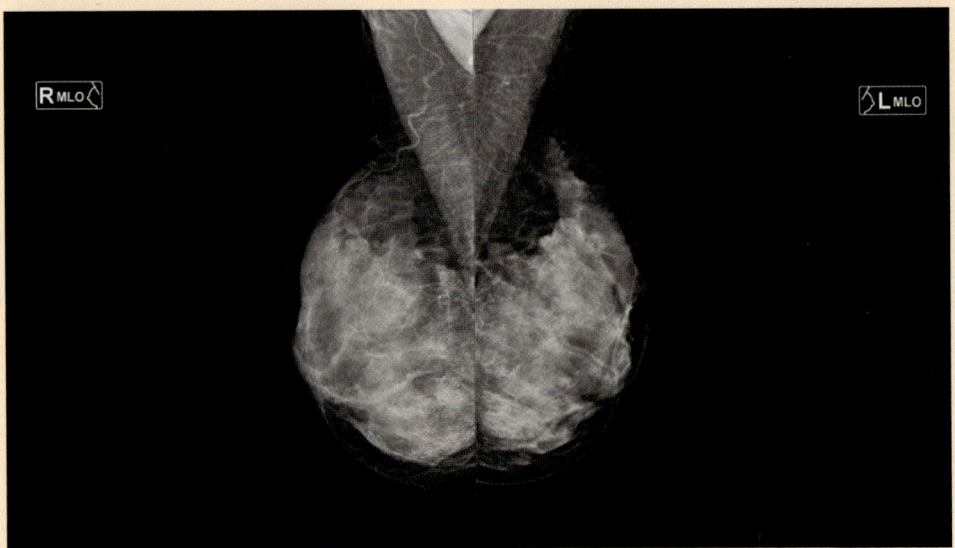

Key Points

Most challenging to detect focal lesions in the background of extremely dense attenuation of breast parenchyma. Small focal lesions are often obscured by the density of normal breast parenchyma. Clinical details including the location of any clinically palpable abnormality should be noted and use of additional modalities (USG, MRI) may be required, if mammography findings do not explain the clinical symptoms.

Routine screening mammography: Incidental benign calcifications

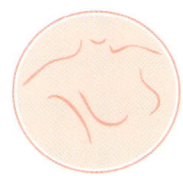

Mammography

ACR Type B density: Multiple tiny benign nodular macrocalcifications, many showing central internal lucency (likely benign cutaneous calcifications). Right mediolateral oblique (MLO) view shows a tiny annular calcification along the skin outline in the upper quadrant BIRADS II, confirming its cutaneous location.

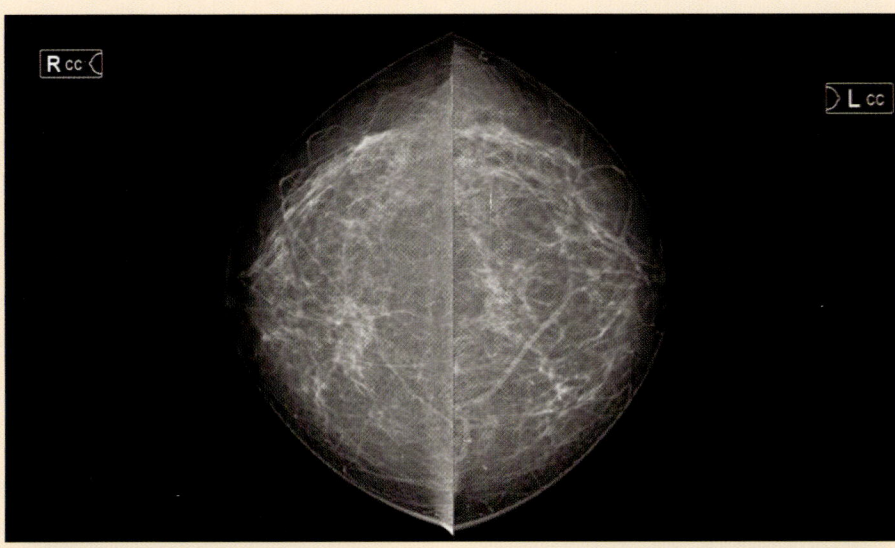

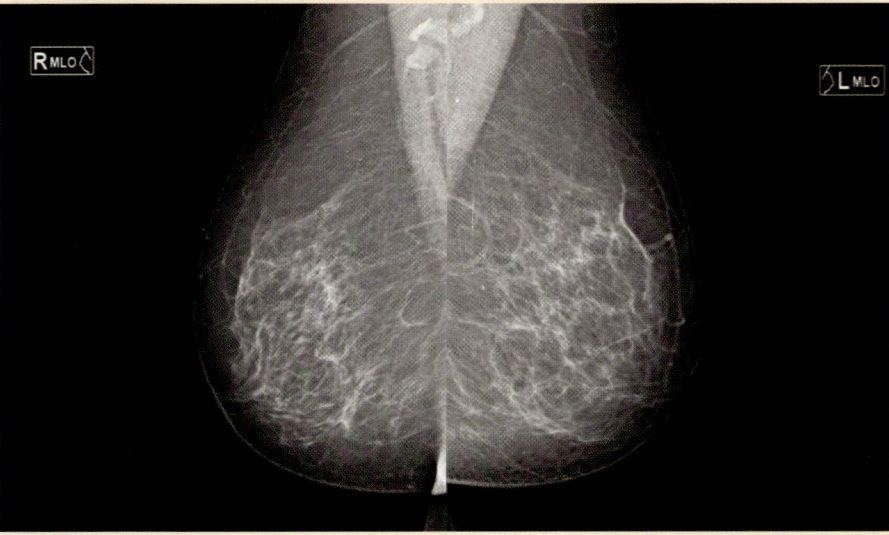

Key Points

It is common to see these 'incidental' benign calcifications in mammograms. These are benign and do not require any further evaluation or follow-up.

Routine screening 6 months after treatment for left breast cancer

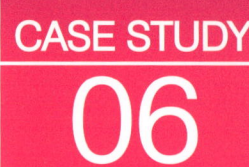
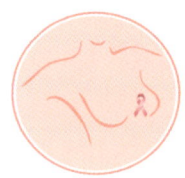

Mammography

History: Ca left breast, post-BCS, post-RT.

Findings:

Both breasts show ACR type B density.

Post-op, post-RT changes seen in left breast with diffuse skin thickening, mild architectural distortion and diffuse stromal thickening.

No spiculated mass or clustered microcalcification seen.

No enlarged axillary nodes seen.

Impression:

Right breast : BIRADS I.

Left breast : BIRADS II.

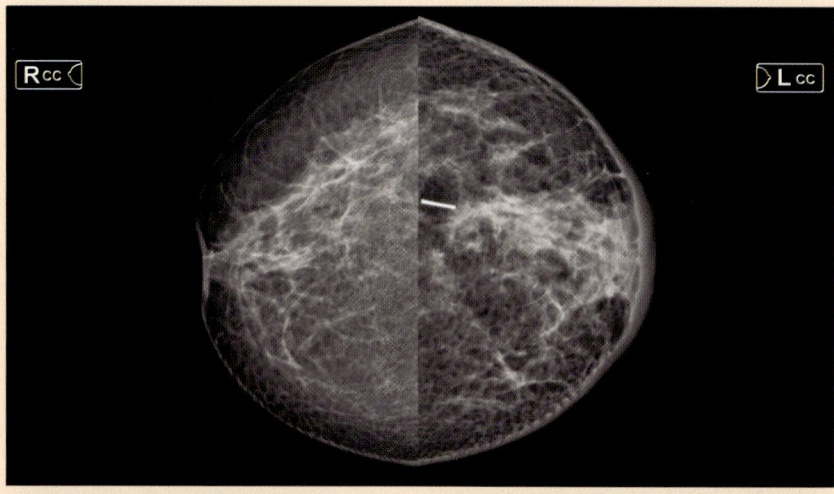

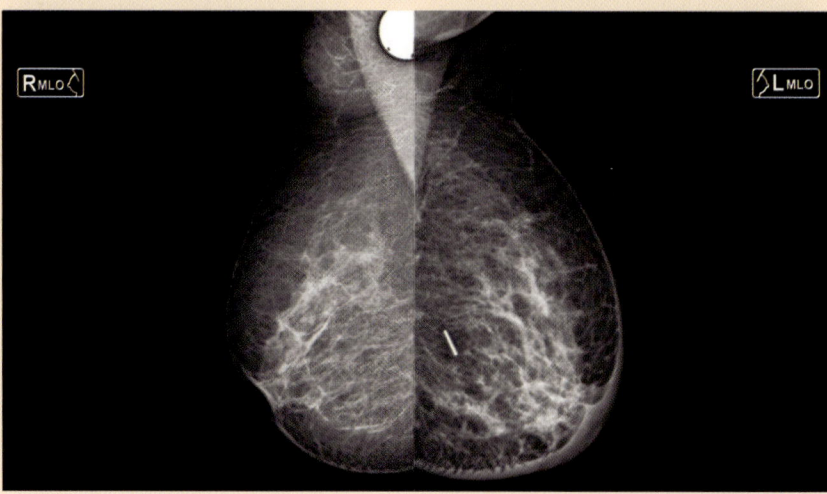

Key Points

Post-treatment (surgery, RT) changes in breast include architectural distortion, scarring, dystrophic calcifications, increased stromal density, skin thickening. Surgical clips may be seen. Rounded opacity of chemoport may be projected over axilla as in this case on right side. Details of treatment should be entered in the mammography requisition form.

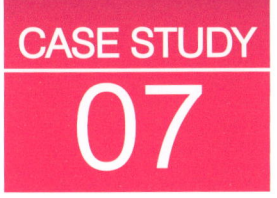

Screening mammography of left breast, post-MRM for Ca left breast

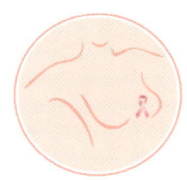

Mammography

Findings: Left breast shows scattered fibroglandular tissue (type 2 density).

There is presence of a focal oval lesion showing popcorn calcification in upper inner quadrant, likely involuting fibroadenoma.

No evidence of any spiculated mass lesion or micro-calcification seen.

No evidence of enlarged axillary nodes seen.

Impression: BIRADS II

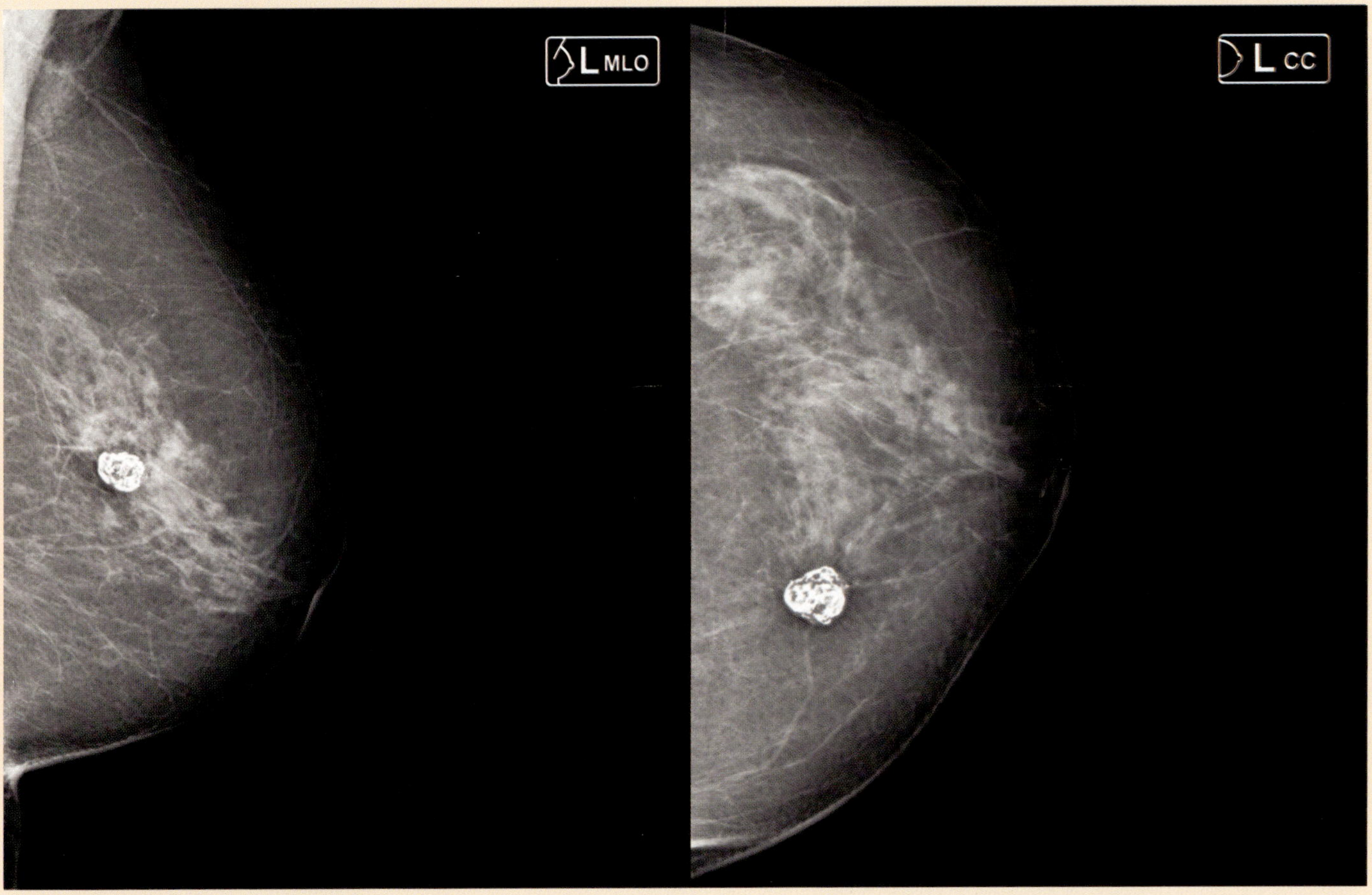

Key Points

This is a typical 'popcorn' calcification in an involuting fibroadenoma.

Routine screening mammography: Incidental vascular calcifications

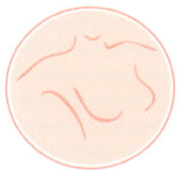

Mammography

ACR Type A density: Extensive vascular calcifications. No abnormal breast parenchymal region. BIRADS I.

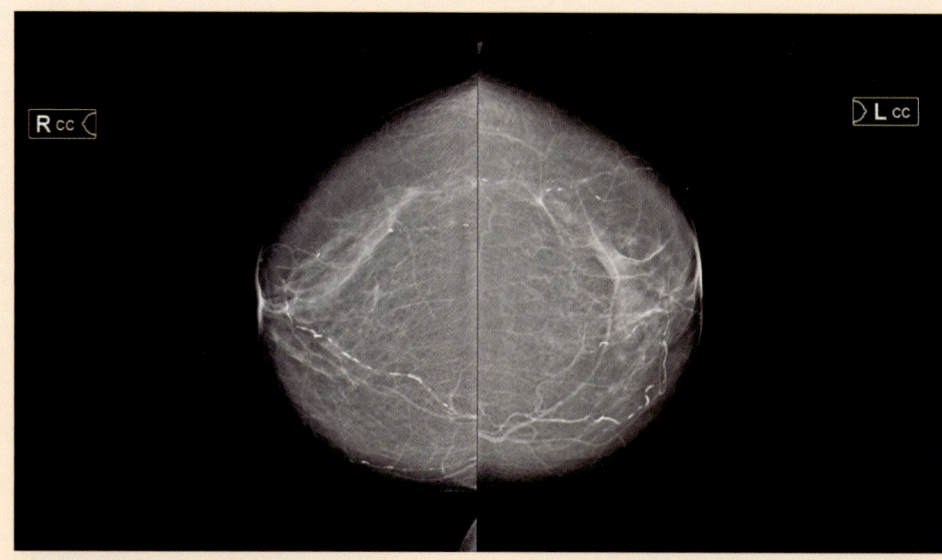

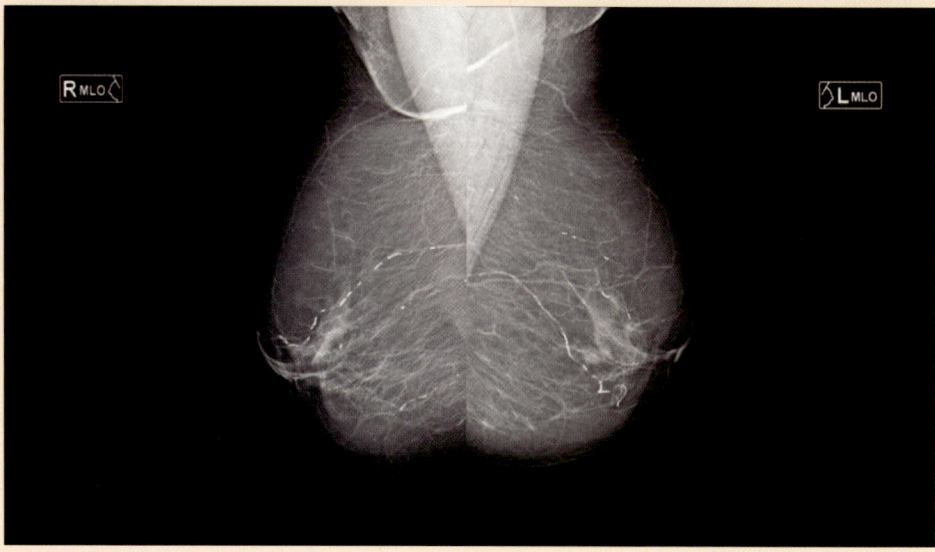

Key Points

It is common to see extensive vascular calcifications, especially in older patients. These should not be confused with breast parenchymal calcifications. Vascular calcifications are curvilinear, remain parallel in orientation and are not in ductal distribution.

65-year-old lady having occasional nipple discharge for last 5 years

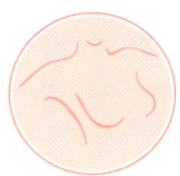

Mammography

ACR Type B density: Thick dense, linear, rod-like large calcifications with smooth margins along with a few tiny nodular macrocalcifications in both breasts, most marked in inferior inner quadrant of right breast. Tubular soft-tissue opacities in inferior, medial quadrant of right breast, in ductal pattern consistent with dilated ducts.

No significant interval changes in comparison to previous mammography studies done one and three years earlier. Findings are consistent with ductal ectasia. BIRADS III. Suggested USG breast correlation and follow-up.

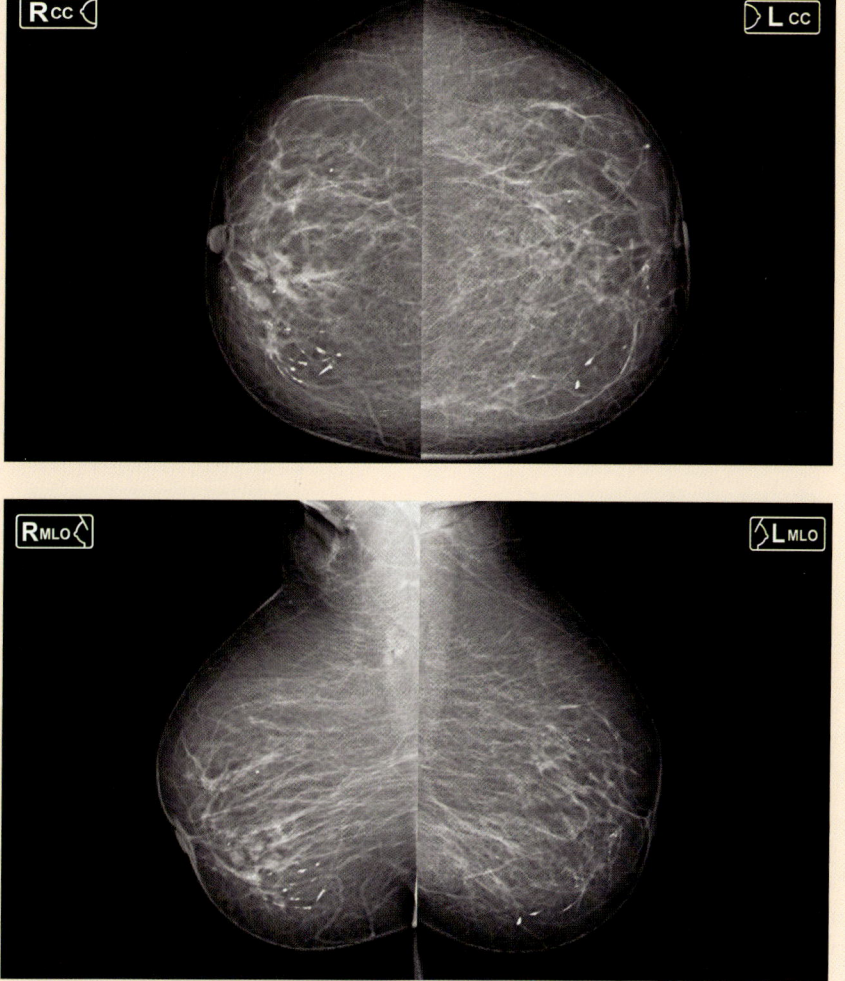

Key Points

Duct ectasia, also called periductal mastitis, comedo mastitis, plasma cell mastitis and mastitis obliterans, is characterized by chronic inflammatory changes leading to clogged debris in dilated ducts. On mammography, the dilated ducts are seen as tubular branching opacities, coursing/converging towards nipple. Calcifications are typically high density rod-/cigar-shaped with smooth outline pointing towards nipple as in this case.

70-year-old lady presenting with right axillary lump

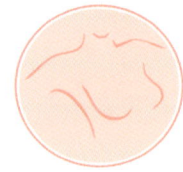

Mammography

ACR Type B density:

No spiculated mass or architectural distortion or clustered microcalcification in either breast.

Mildly enlarged (2 cm in short axis) and a few sub-centiemeter dense right axillary nodes.

BIRADS I, Further evaluation of right axillary nodes by FNAC suggested.

FNAC right axillary node shows cellular smear with lymphoid cells in various stages of maturation, cosistent with reactive lymphadenitis.

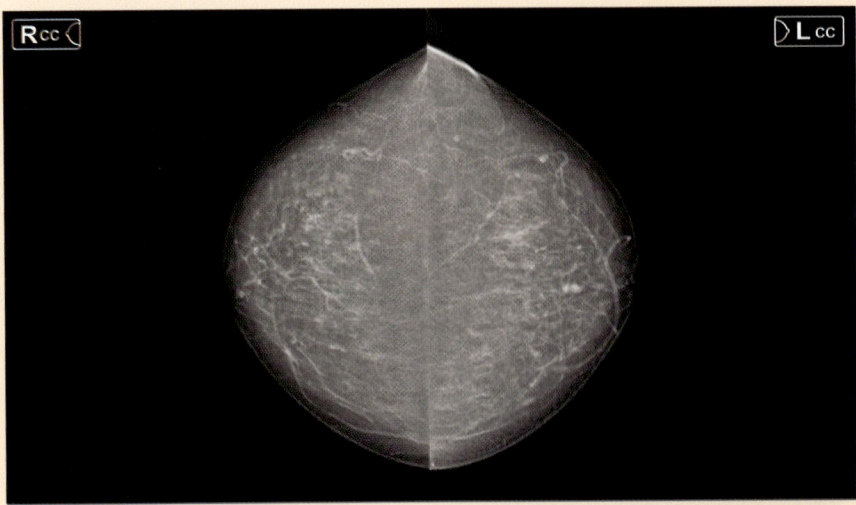

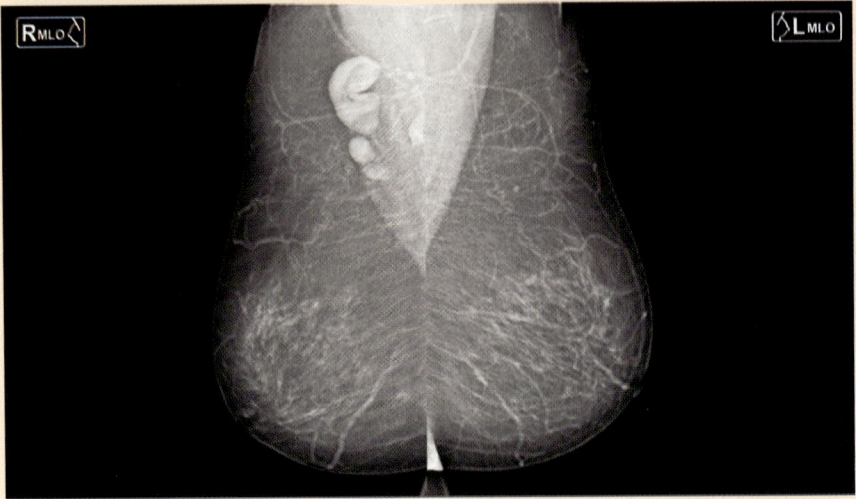

Key Points

It is not uncommon to see a setting of no abnormality on mammography with unilateral enlarged axillary nodes. USG-guided FNA/biopsy can quickly establish the etiology of enlarged nodes. Further breast evaluation by MRI can be done, if the node FNA/biopsy raises concern for a breast primary.

71-year-old lady, post left MRM for Ca breast with right breast lumpectomy for benign lesion

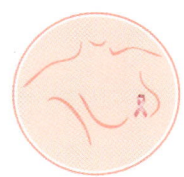

Mammography

ACR Type C density:

Multiple smooth marginated round to oval soft tissue lesions, some showing internal coarse calcification. No spiculated mass/clustered micro-calcifications.

Impression: Findings suggest likely involuting fibroadenomas (BIRADS III). Suggested follow-up mammography at 6 months.

USG breast shows smooth marginated oval hypoechoic lesions with internal calcifications and mild posterior acoustic enhancement.

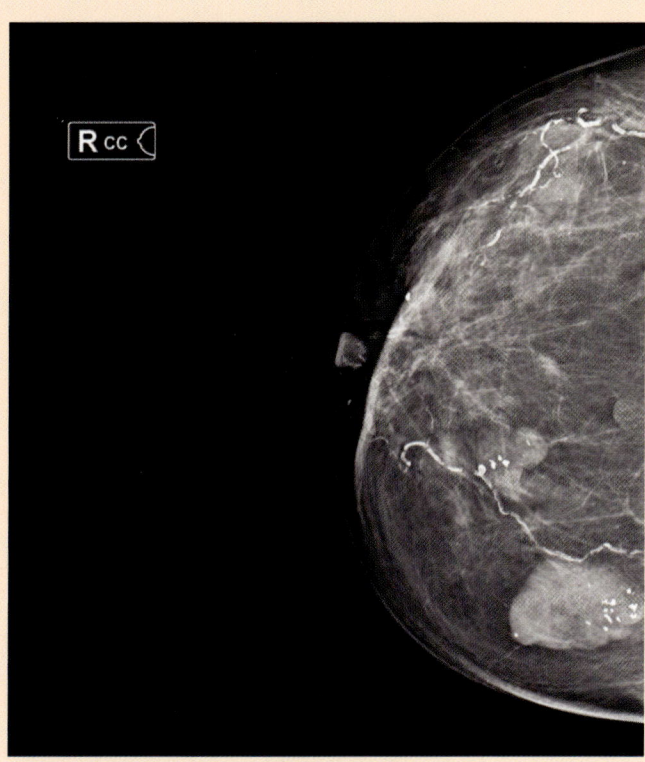
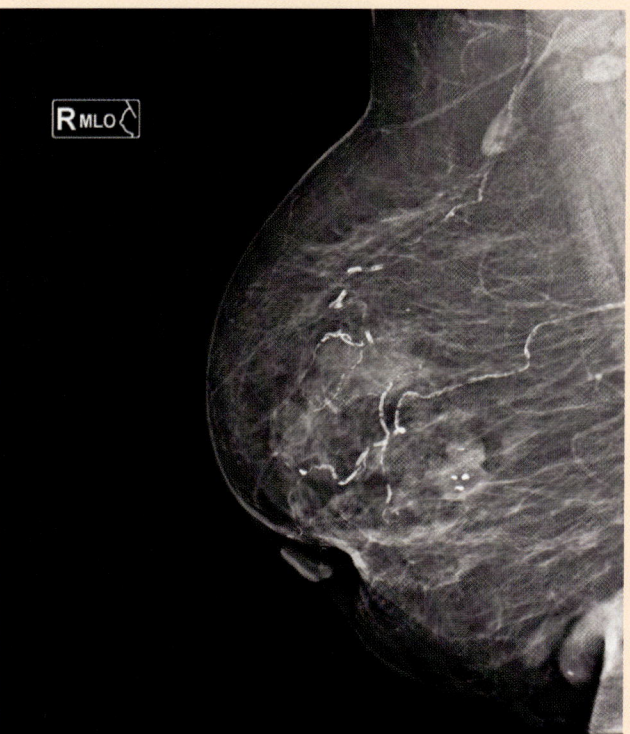

Key Points

Focal breast lesions appearing to be likely benign, BIRADS III, need to be followed by 3 to 6 monthly mammography or ultrasound. Alternatively, HPE correlation can be done by USG-guided/surgical excision biopsy.

61-year-old lady with history of right breast lumpectomy for benign lesion 5 months back

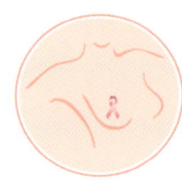

Mammography

ACR Type A density.

Postoperative changes with mild architectural distortion and skin puckering in right breast. Smooth marginated rounded opacity of 7 cm in upper outer quadrant of right breast at the operative site. Findings suggest likely postoperative seroma/ collection, which requires USG correlation.

USG breast: Thin-walled cyst in the right breast corresponding to the lesion seen on mammography with no discenrnible solid intramural component. BIRADS II.

The collection was drained surgically.

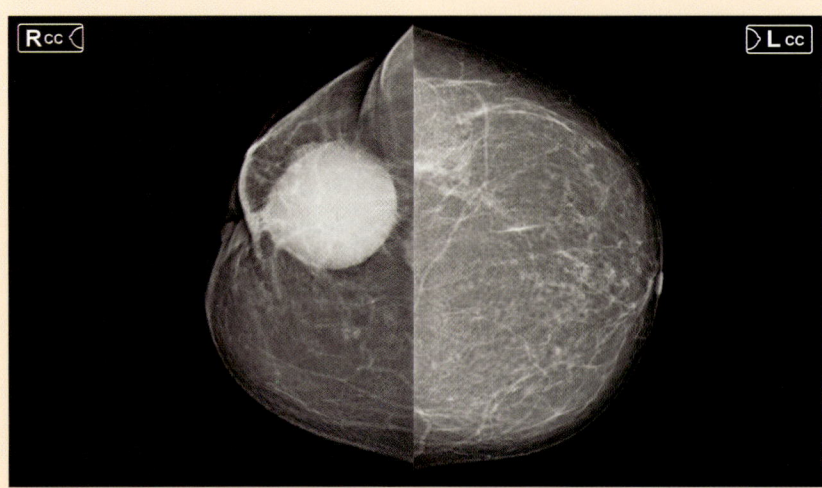

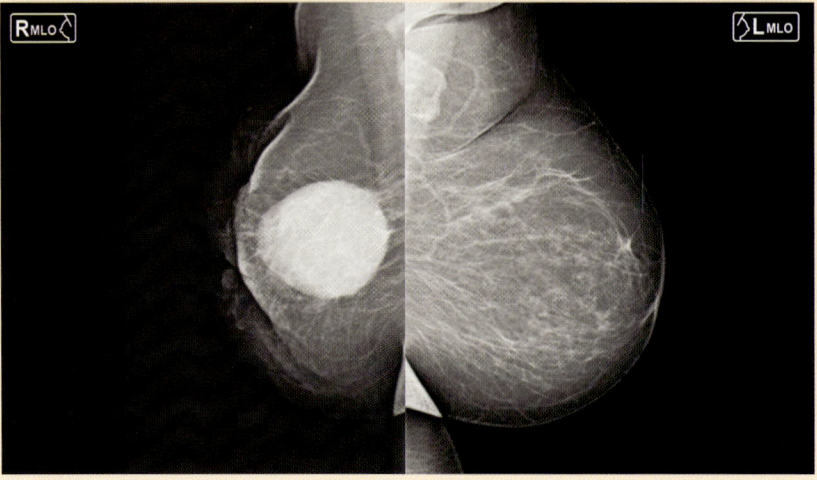

Key Points

Smooth marginated opacity at the operative site in the first postoperative follow-up mammogram (generally done 6 months after surgery) in the absence of any clinical suspicion of recurrent mass with adequate HPE documented surgical excision is typical of a postoperative seroma. These can appear to be denser than simple cysts, due to internal hemorrhagic contents. USG should be suggested for confirmation and to exclude any possible suspicious solid component.

70-year-old lady presenting with bilateral breast discomfort

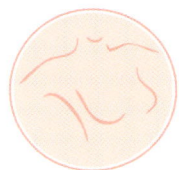

Mammography

ACR Type A density: Small nodular macrocalcifications in upper outer quadrant of right breast with no other focal lesion or architectural distortion or any clustered microcalcification. BIRADS II.

Note made of clustered multiple subcentimeter and enlarged bilateral axillary nodes. Needs further evaluation.

PET-CT done for further evaluation revealed cervical, bilateral axillary and retroperitoneal lymphadenopathy with hypermetabolic nasopharyngeal, tonsillar lesion.

HPE: Non-Hodgkin's lymphoma

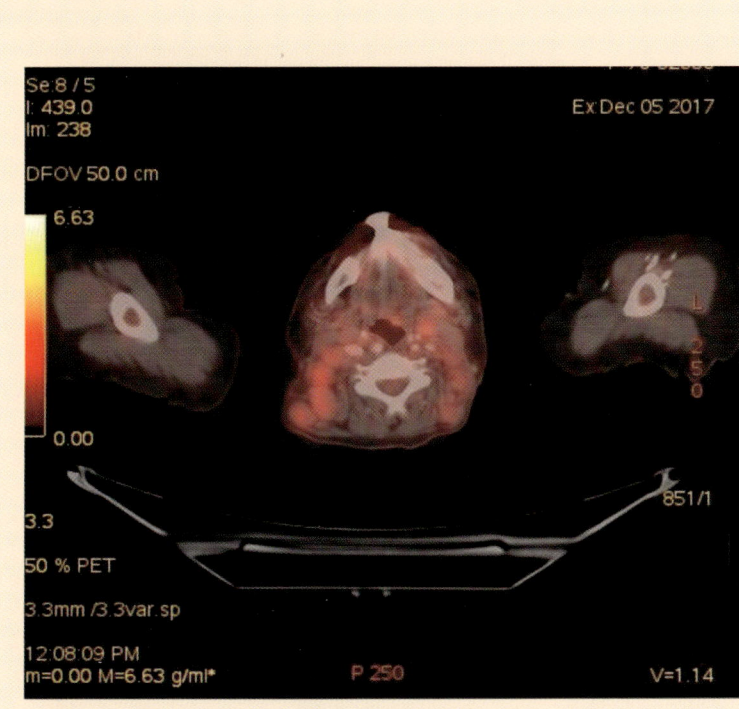

PET-CT Image

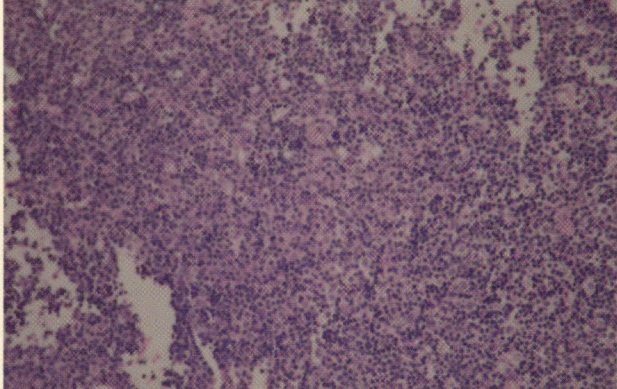

H&E 40x atypical small lymphoid cells

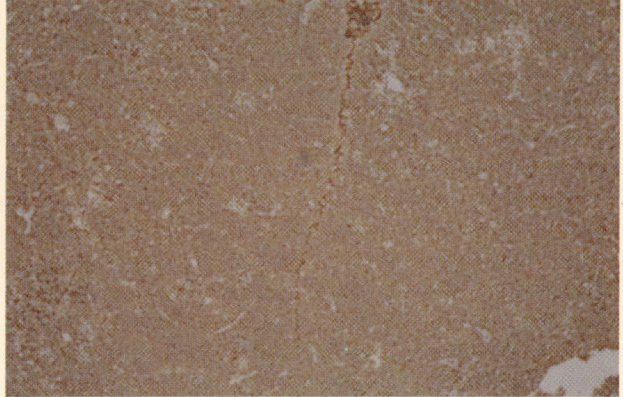

IHC CD5 B-CLL

Key Points

Bilateral symmetric axillary lymphadenopathy in the absence of any mammography detectable suspicious breast lesion is unlikely to be related to any breast abnormality. Further evaluation with whole body imaging and lymph node biopsy would help to know the etiology and extent of disease.

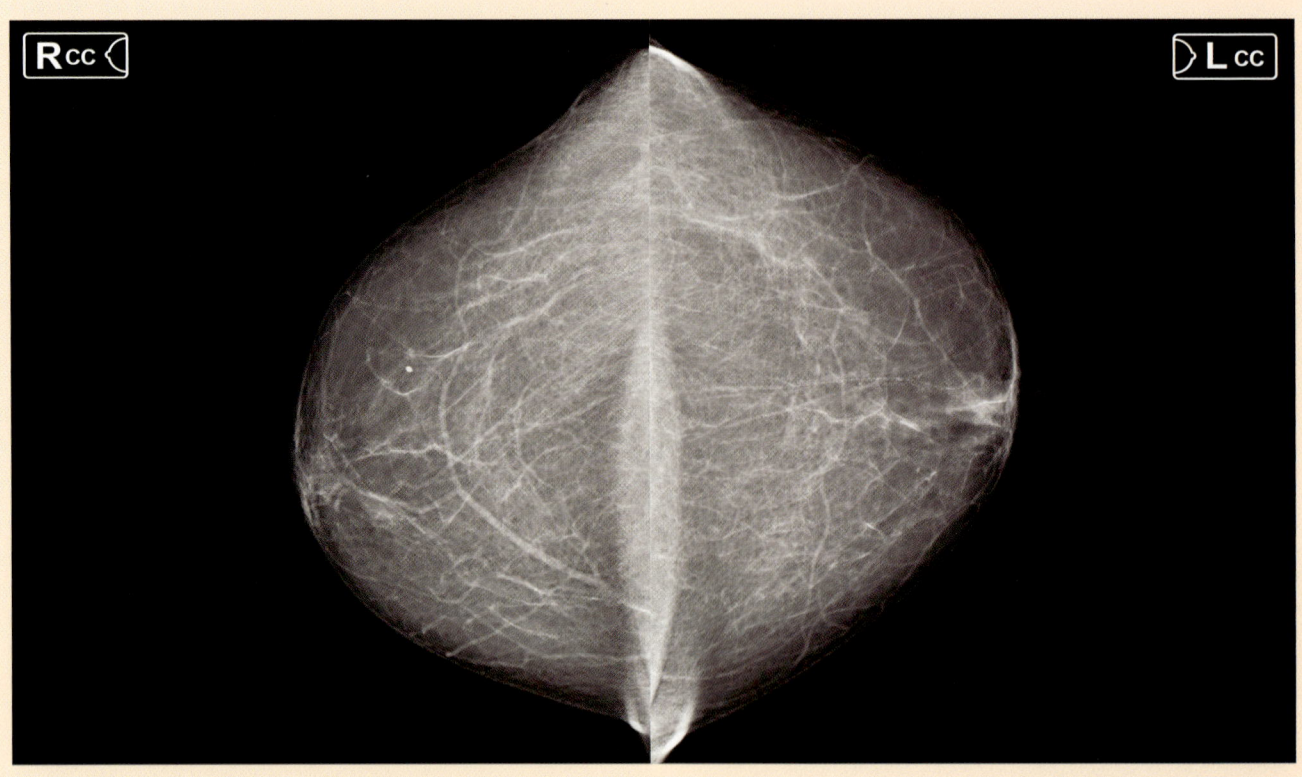

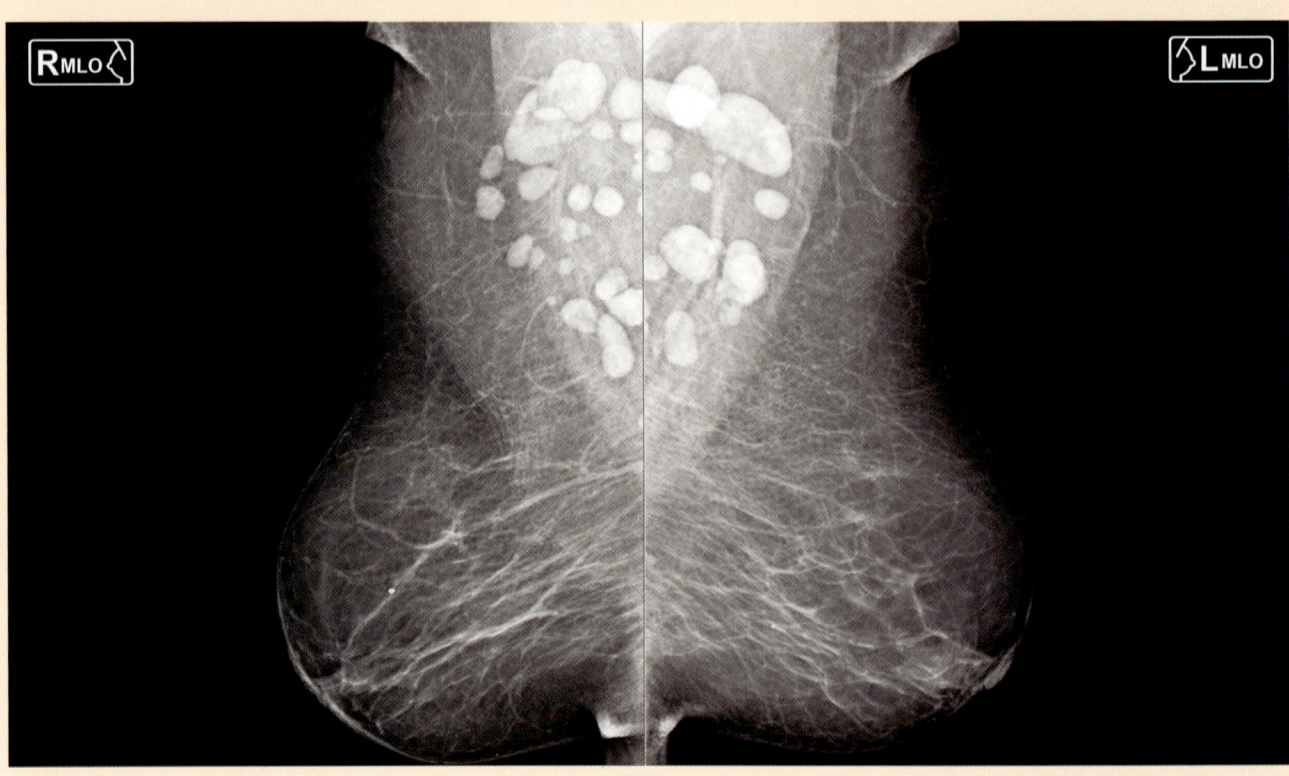

40-year-old lady presenting with lump in left breast for last 10 days

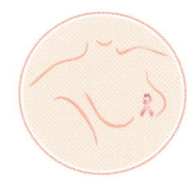

Mammography

ACR Type C density: Area of asymmetric density in the inferior, outer quadrant of left breast.

No significant abnormality in the right breast.

BIRADS 0.

Further evaluation by USG ± FNAC suggeted.

USG breast revealed a small irregular lesion of size 1.3 x 1.1 cm with surrounding architectural distortion in left breast at 5 O'clock position.

USG-guided FNAC was positive for breast carcinoma.

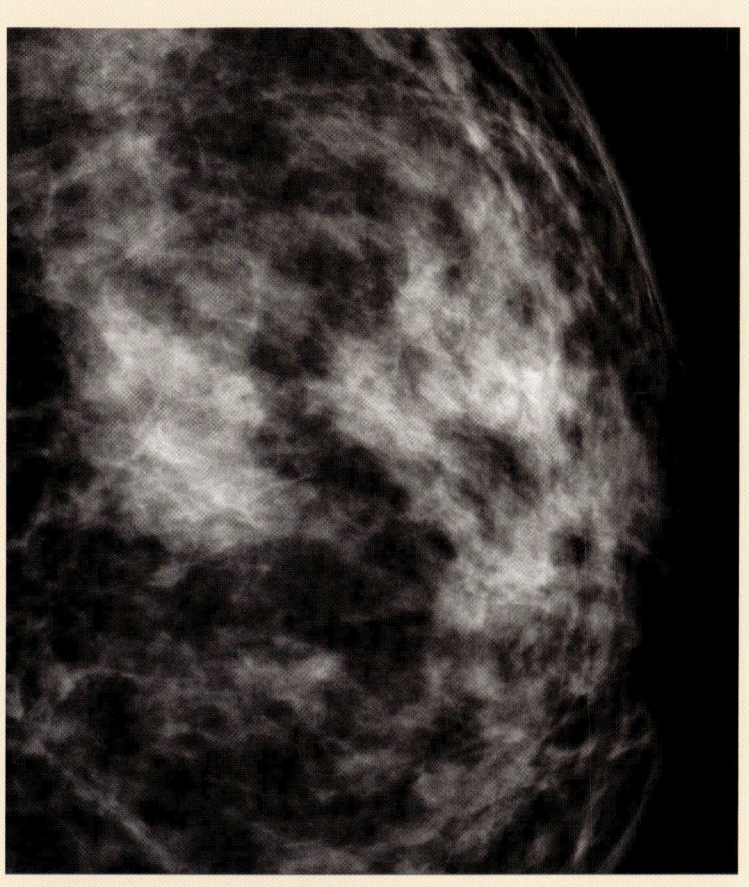

Zoomed left CC image

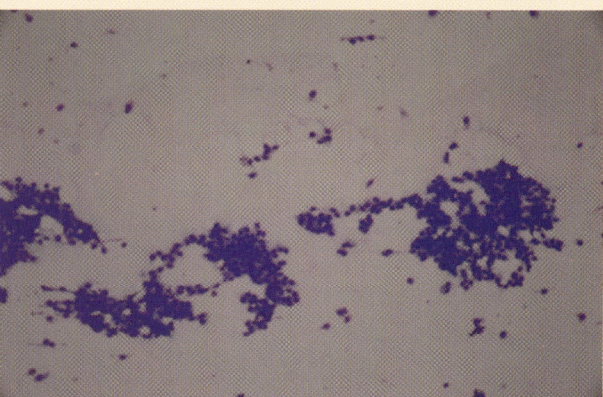

FNAC image

Key Points

Many cancers are seen as areas of asymmetric density on mammogram. All focal asymmetric densities should be reported and evaluated further to conclusion. Not all asymmetric densities are pathological, but further evaluation with USG, MRI needs to be done to exclude any underlying sinister lesion.

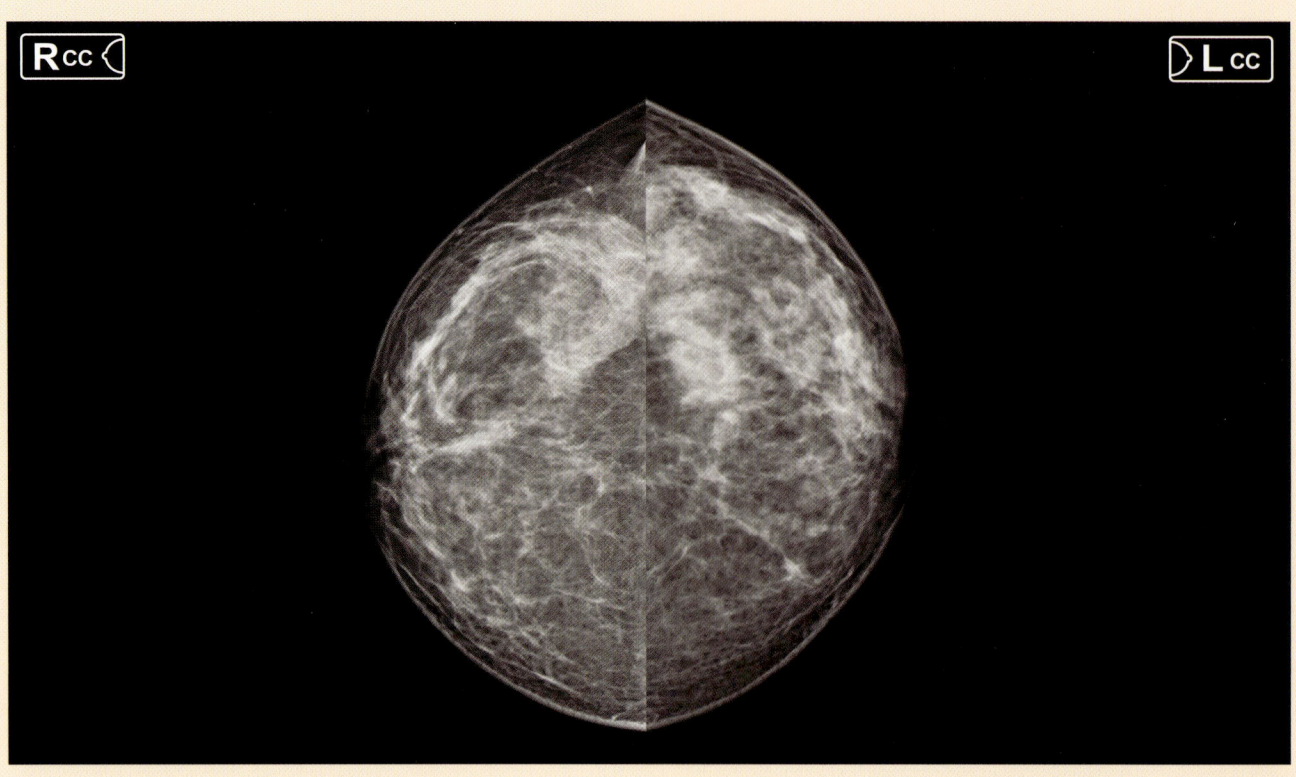

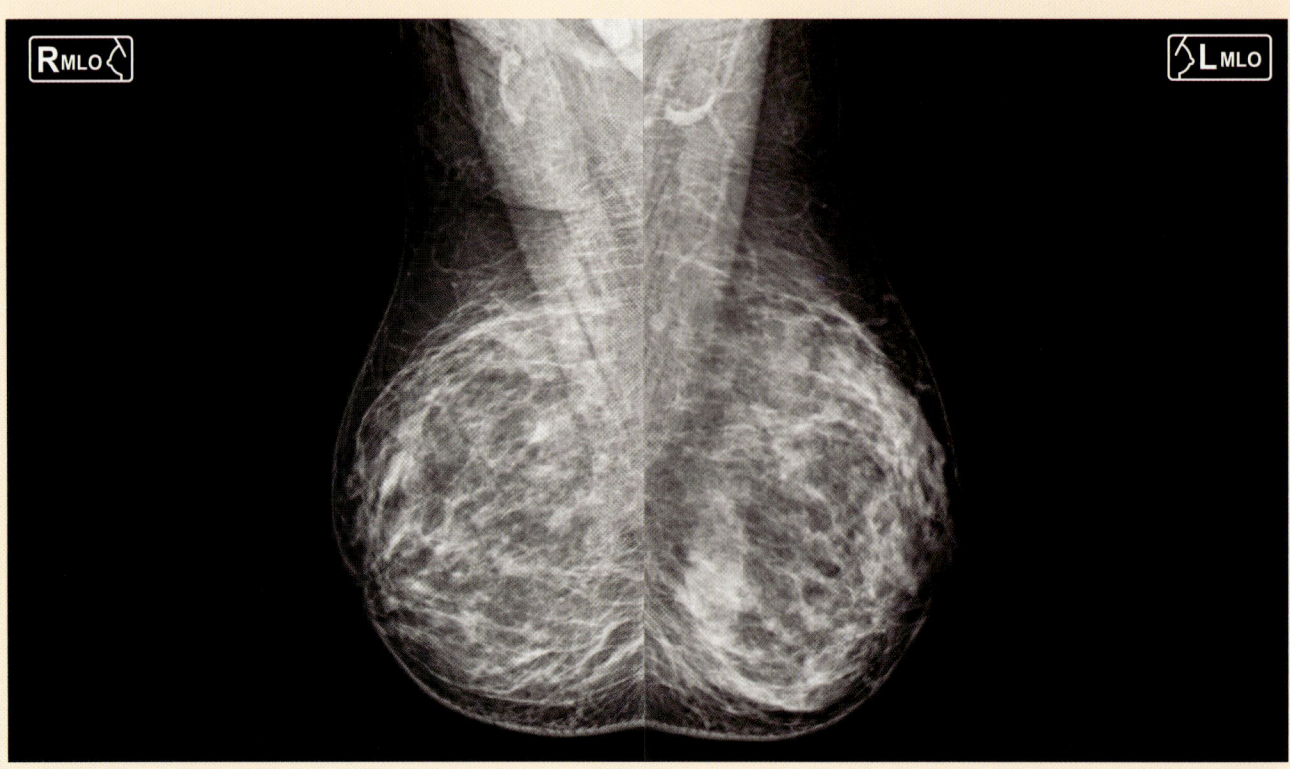

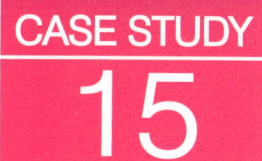

CASE STUDY 15

Screening mammography: Incidental benign cysts

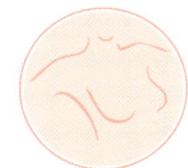

Mammography

ACR Type B density.

Multiple small smooth marginated faint opacities scattered in both breasts.

No spiculated mass at architectural distortion or clustered microcalcification seen.

BIRADS III.

USG correlation suggested.

USG breast reveals multiple small subcentimeter thin-walled cysts of varying sizes in both breasts with no solid intramural component in any of the cysts. USG BIRADS II.

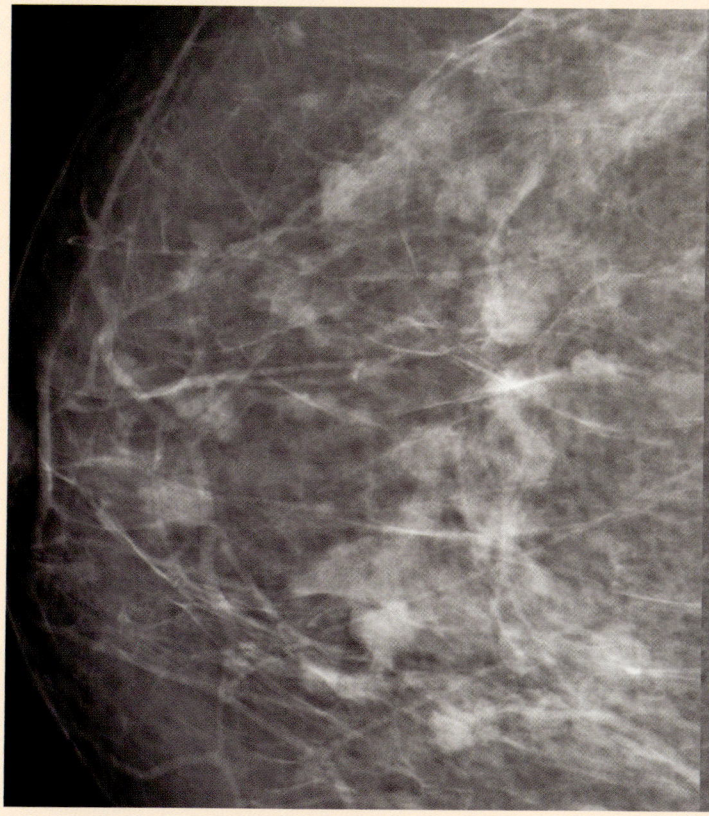

Zoomed right CC image

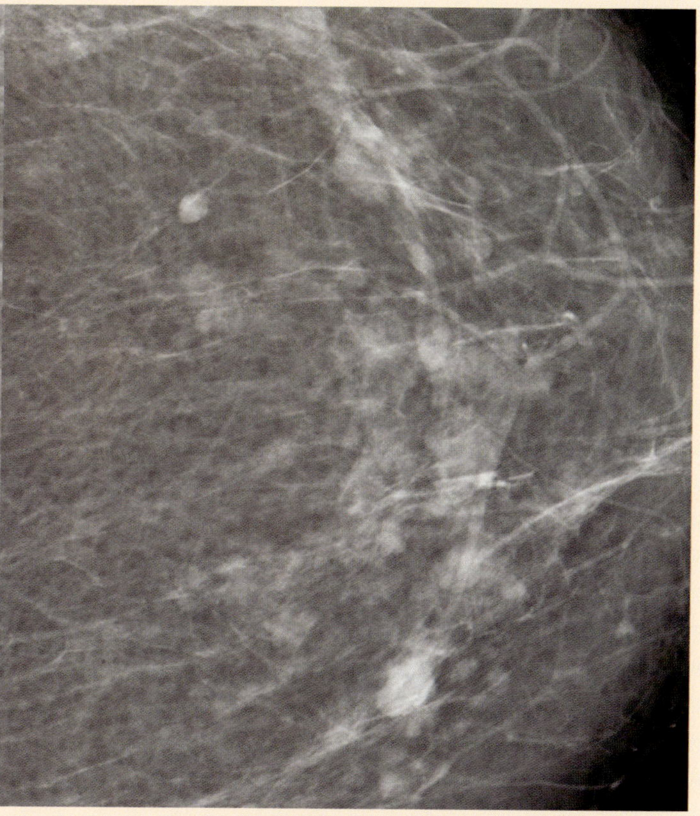

Zoomed left CC image

Key Points

Benign cysts have faint opacity unlike most solid lesions which are much denser in attenuation. Importantly benign lesions show a smooth outline and show no associated breast architectural distortion. USG should be suggested to confirm mammography findings.

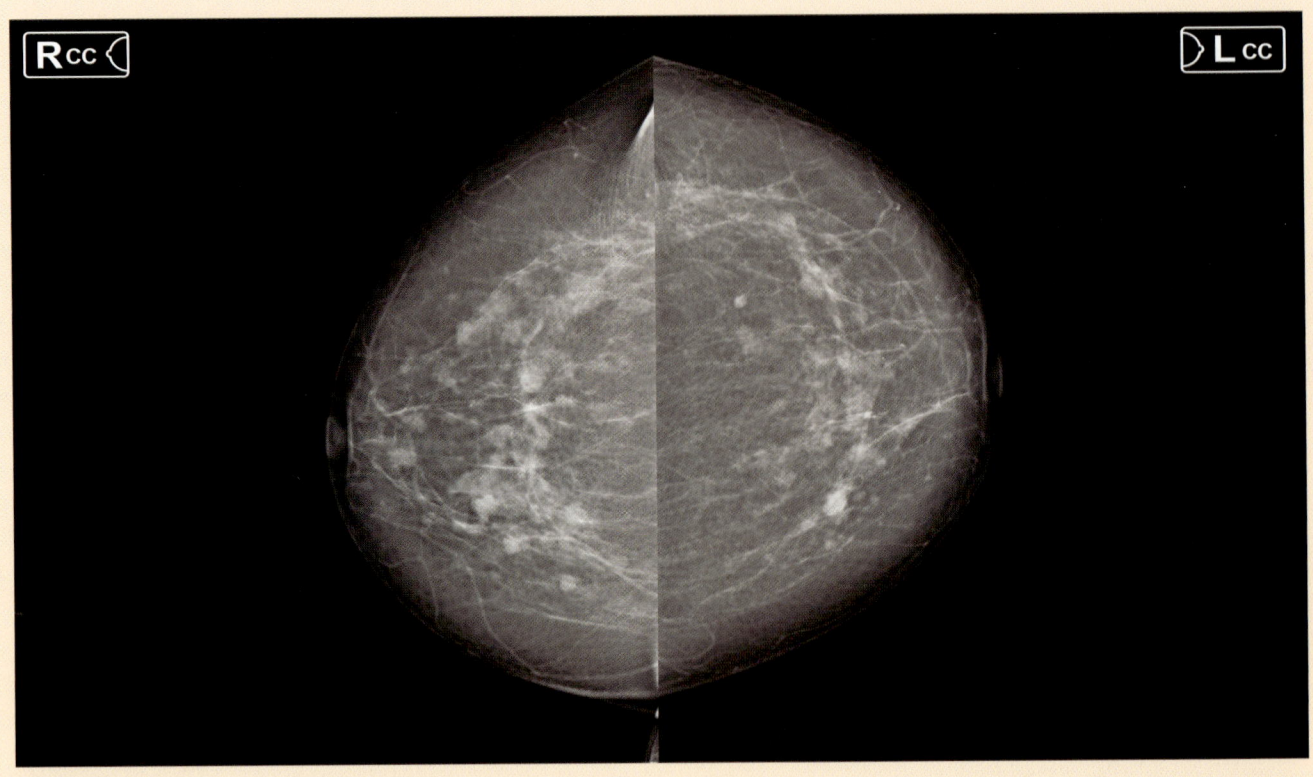

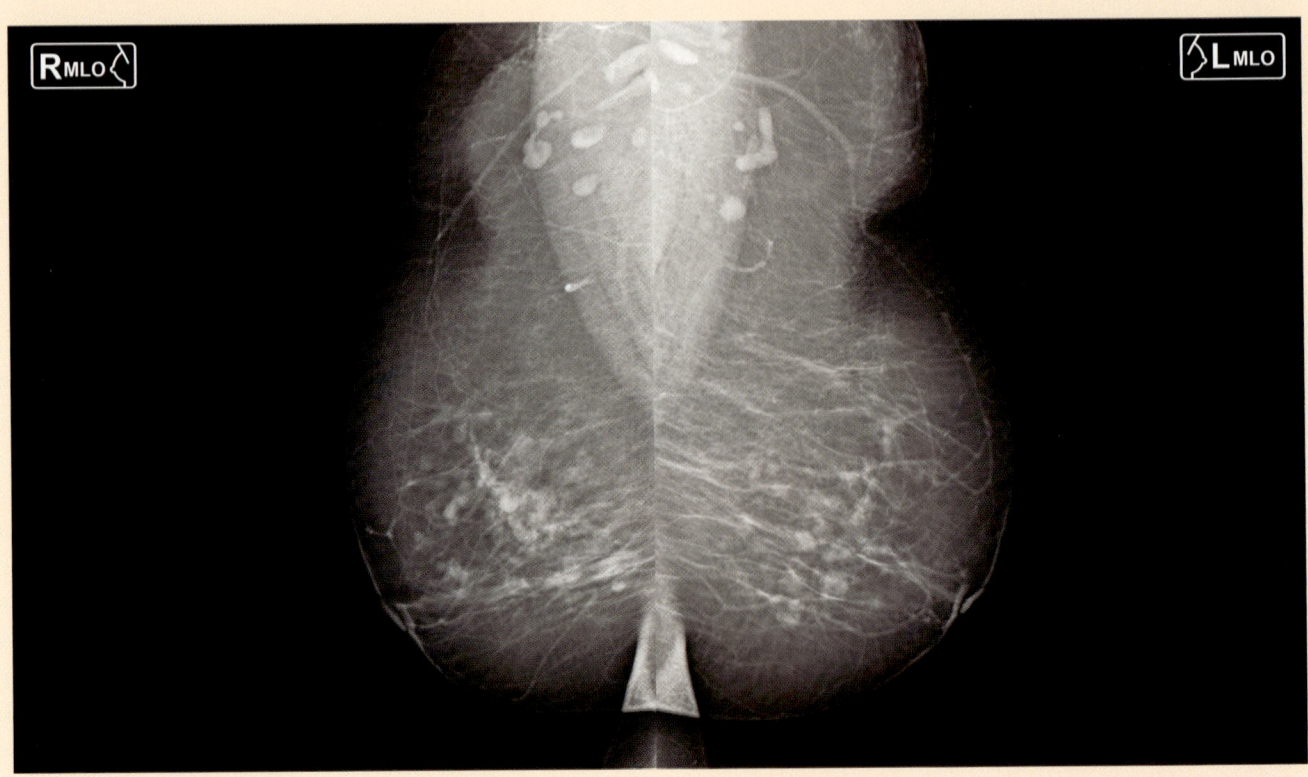

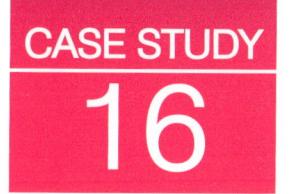

67-year-old lady with right nipple discharge

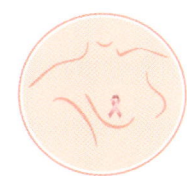

Mammography

ACR Type A density.

Right breast shows a rounded soft tissue density lesion with microlobulations in the retroareolar region.

BIRADS V

USG-guided biopsy: Features sugeestive of adenosis with papilloma.

Right breast lumpectomy HPE reveals intraductal Papillomatosis with foci of usual epithelial hyperplasia.

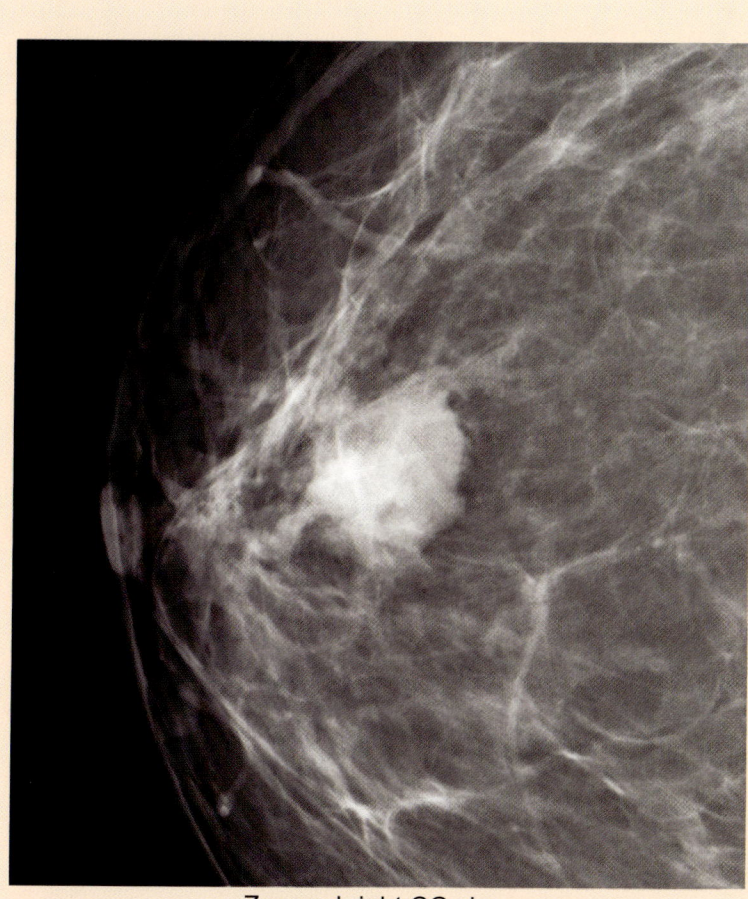

Zoomed right CC view

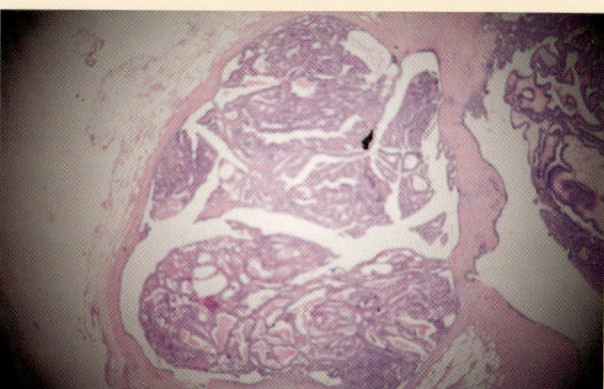

HPE image

Key Points

Rounded mass lesion with microlobulations, detected at this age is suspicious for malignancy. Trucut biopsy was negative, but it is advisable to do an excision biopsy of such lesions since there may be a small focus of malignancy in an otherwise benign lesion and not represented in a trucut biopsy core. In this case, excision biopsy was also negative. The lesion in this case is in the retroareolar region, which is a review area and special attention should be given to exclude a lesion in this location.

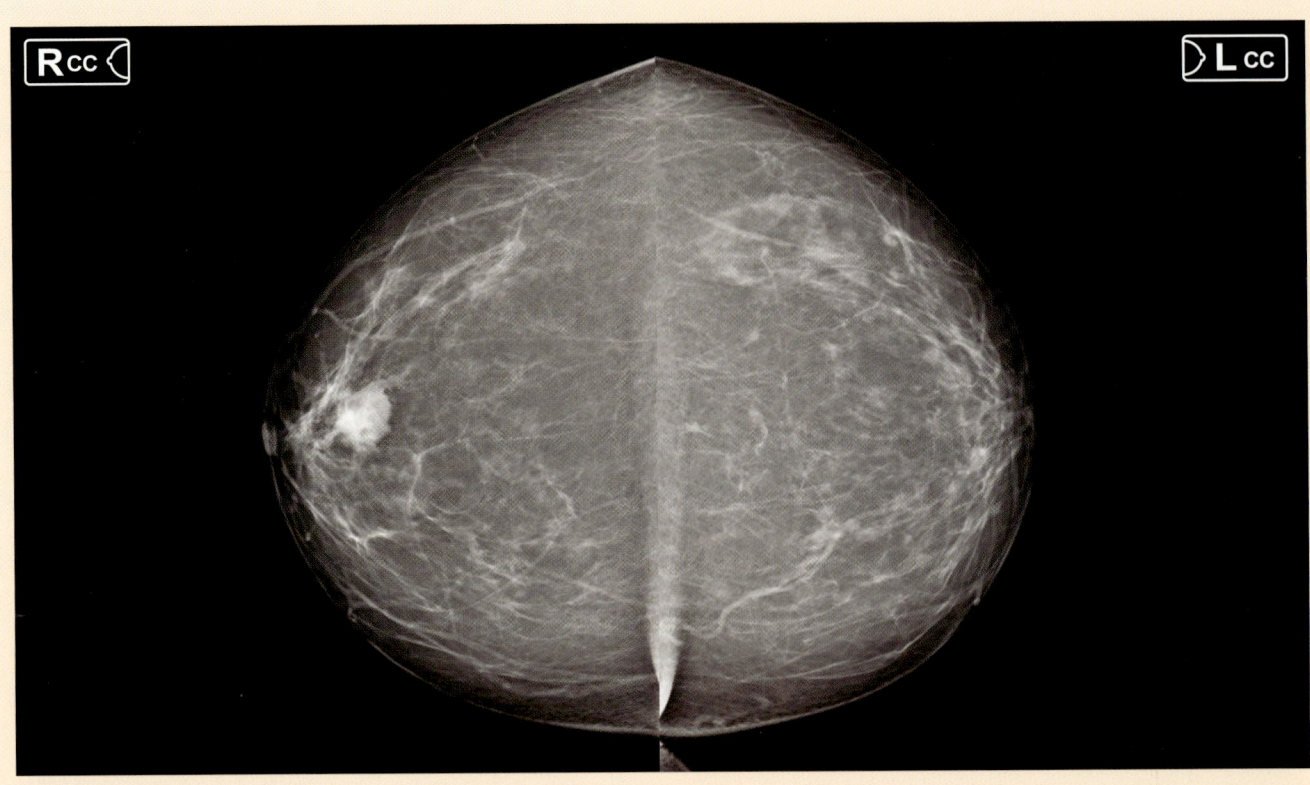

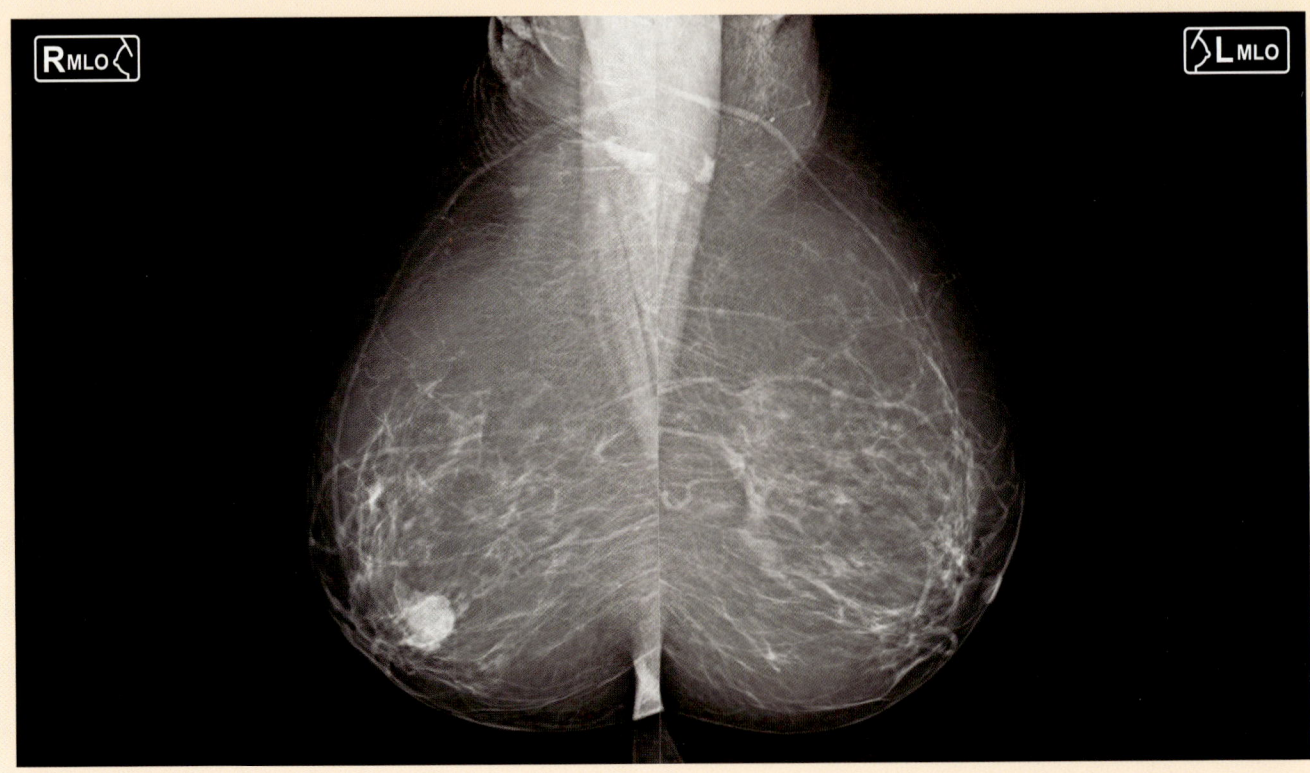

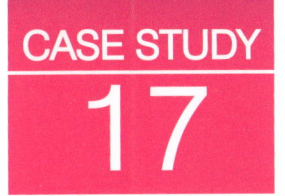

45-year-old lady with lump in right breast

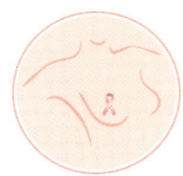

Mammography

ACR Type C density.

Smooth marginated oval opacity of (2.7 x 2.1 cm) in upper quadrant of right breast.

No associated architectural distortion with no internal microcalcifications. BIRADS III.

Suggested USG / FNAC correlation.

FNAC right breast lesion shows cellular smears comprising of slightly cohesive clusters of ductal epithelial cells revealing bland nuclear chromatin. Overall suggest breast cytology code 3 (atypical, probably benign). Excision biopsy suggested by the pathologist.

Excision biopsy HPE: Benign fibroadenoma with foci of sclerosing adenosis, duct ectasia and apocrine metaplasia.

FNAC image

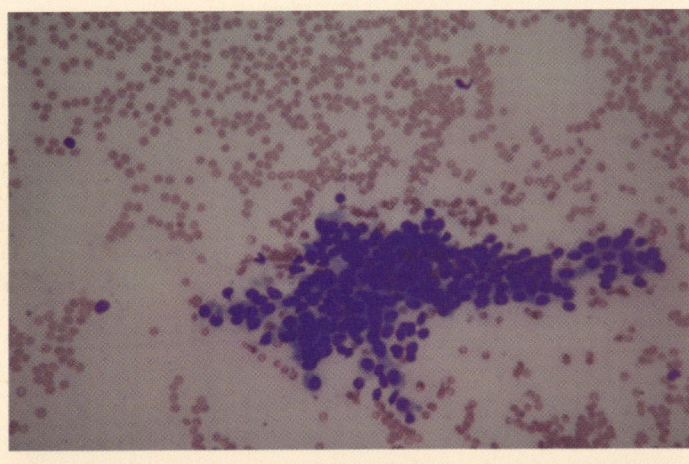

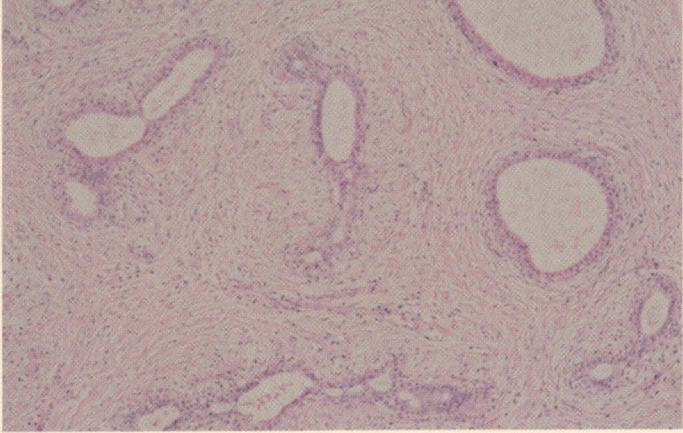

HPE image

Key Points

Solid lesions are generally of the same or higher attenuation than the native breast parenchyma. Smooth margins and oval shape in the absence of associated architectural distortion or internal microcalcifications suggest a likely benign lesion. These lesions need to be followed with a serial mammogram at 3 to 6 months or a USG-guided FNAC/biopsy can be done. In this case, the pathologist raised concerns of atypia in FNAC and suggested excision biopsy which was done. HPE of excision specimen revealed a benign fibroadenoma.

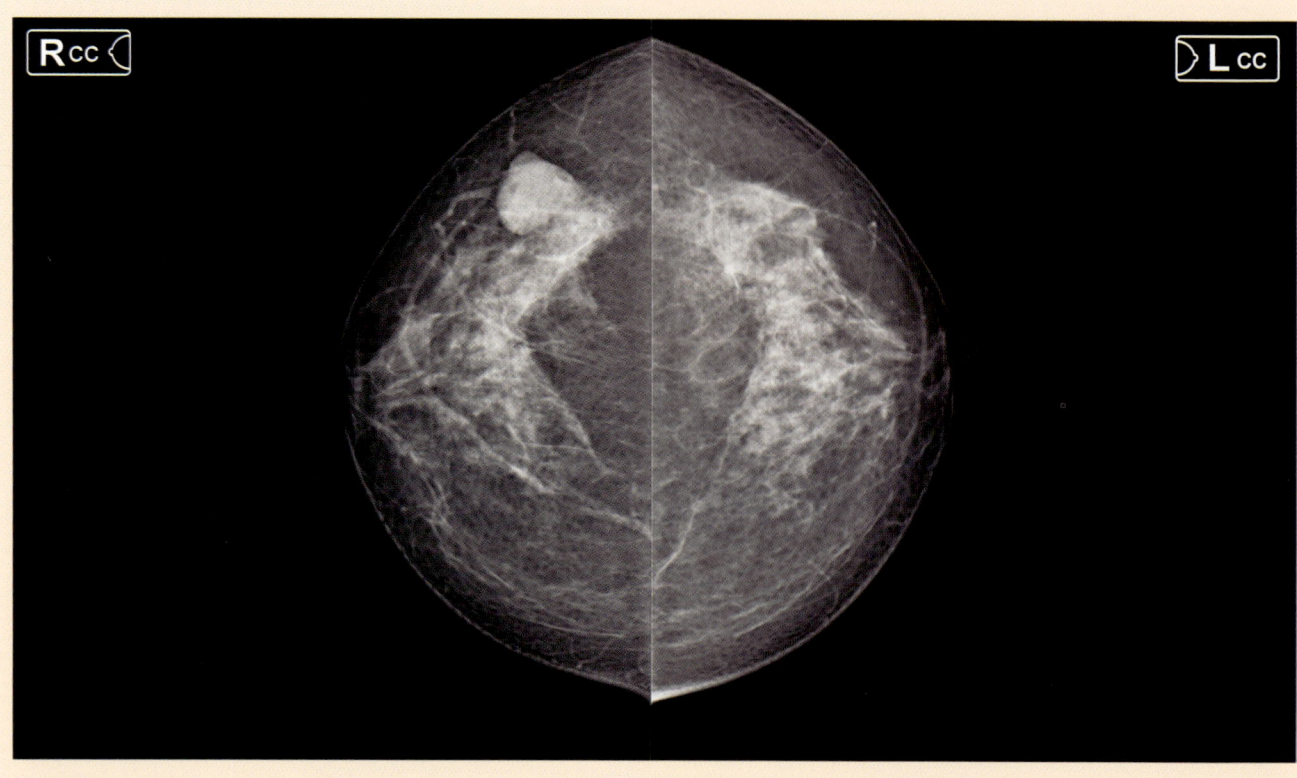

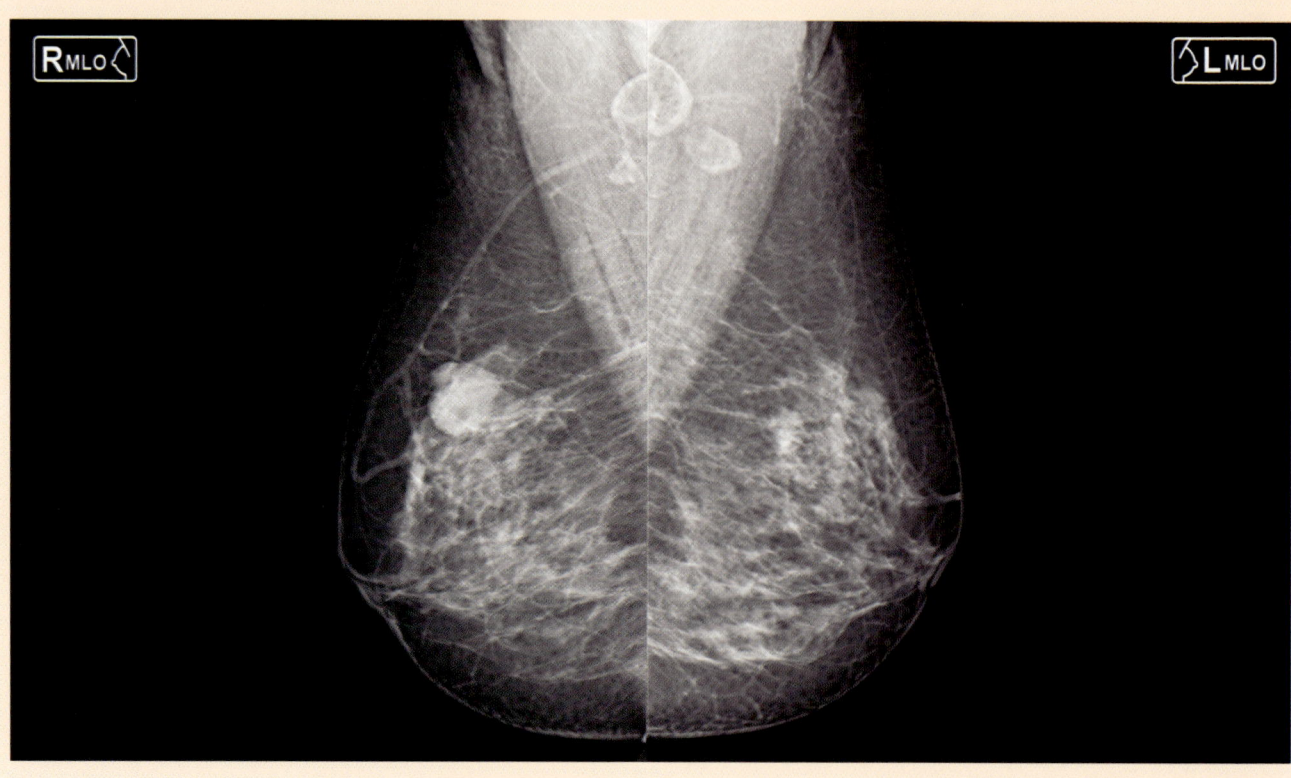

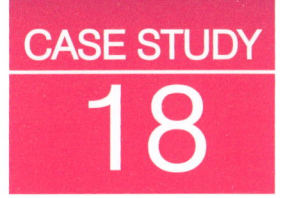

66-year-old lady presenting with lump in left breast

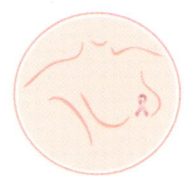

Mammography

ACR Type A density.

Left breast shows a rounded mass (2.1 cm) lesion with irregular margins in inferior, central quadrant .

BIRADS V

USG-guided FNAC: Positive for malignant cells.

MRM specimen HPE: Invasive mammary carcinoma.

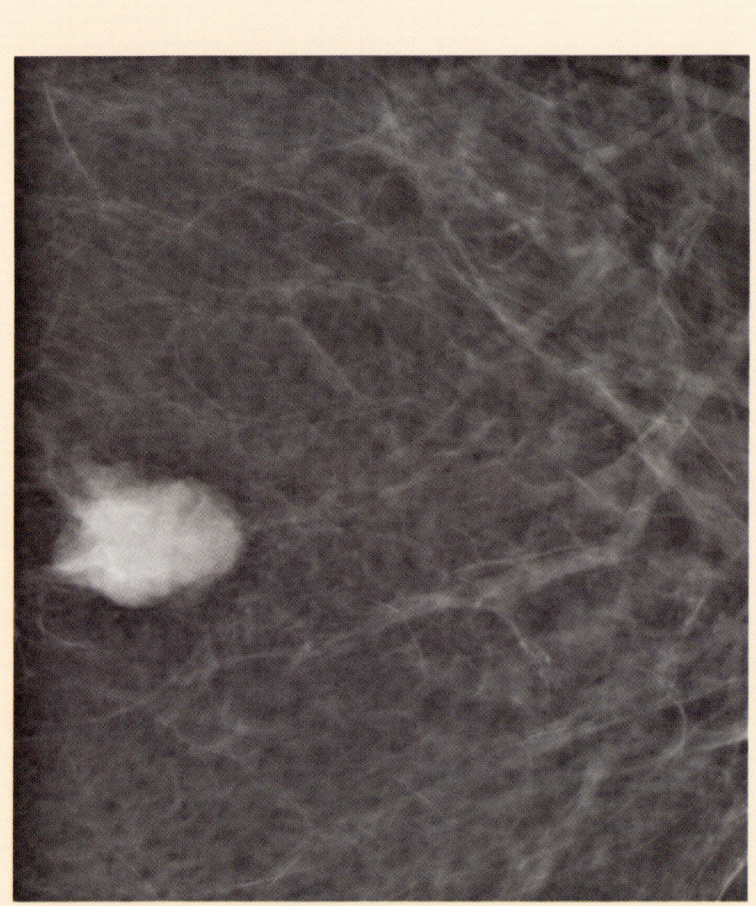

Zoomed left CC view

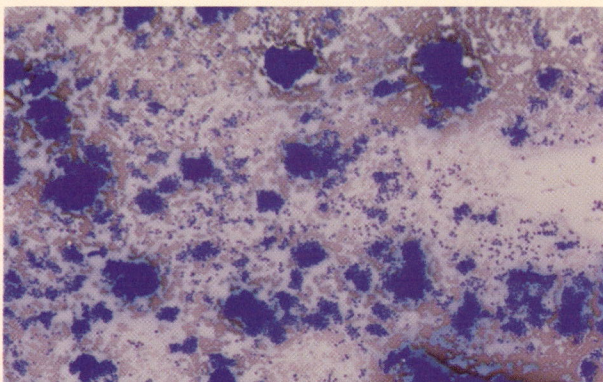

HPE image

Key Points

Spiculated outline in only a small portion of a mass is also highly suspicious for underlying malignant etiology. The lesion is situated in the retromammary area which is a review area and special attention should be given not to miss a lesion in this location.

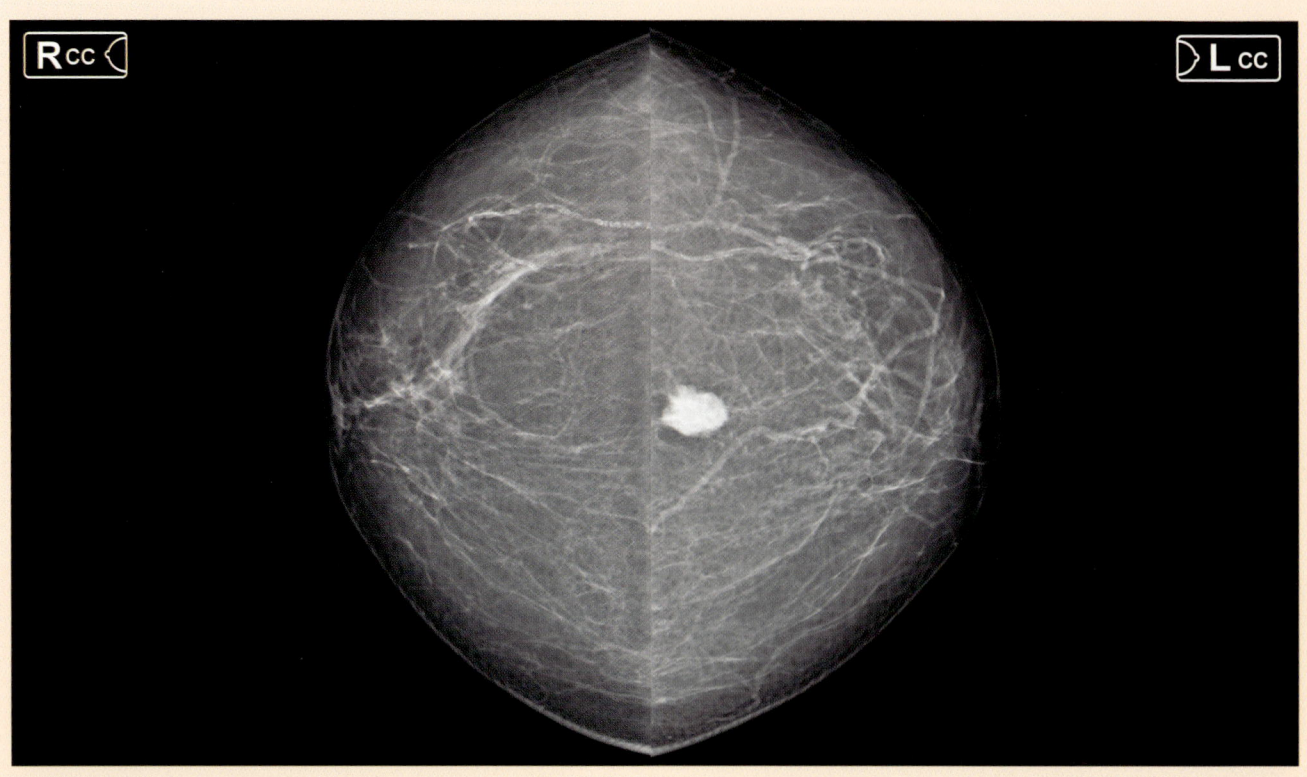

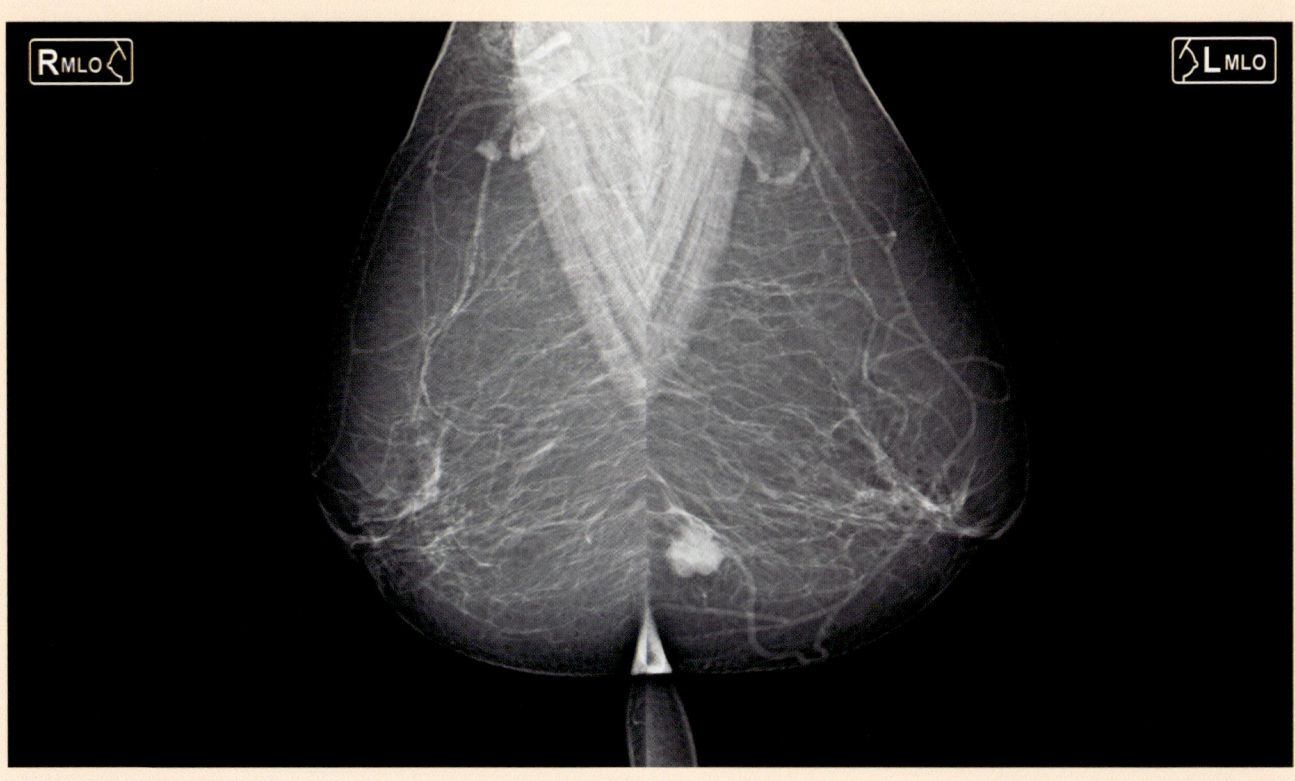

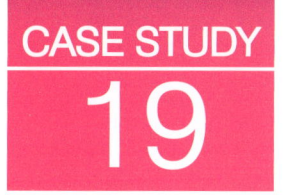

40-year-old lady with lump in right breast

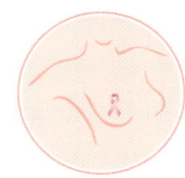

Mammography

ACR Type C density.

Asymmetric density in upper outer quadrant of right breast with no other focal abnormality in either breast. Spot magnification view of right breast abnormality reveals a smooth marginated opacity showing mildly hyperdense differential attenuation.

Ultrasound showed a thin-walled cystic lesion with no discernible solid components.

USG-guided FNAC: Aspirated fluid shows BIRADS III no evidence of malignancy. Monolayered sheet of epithelial cells showing uniform apocrine metaplasia with foaming histiocytes.

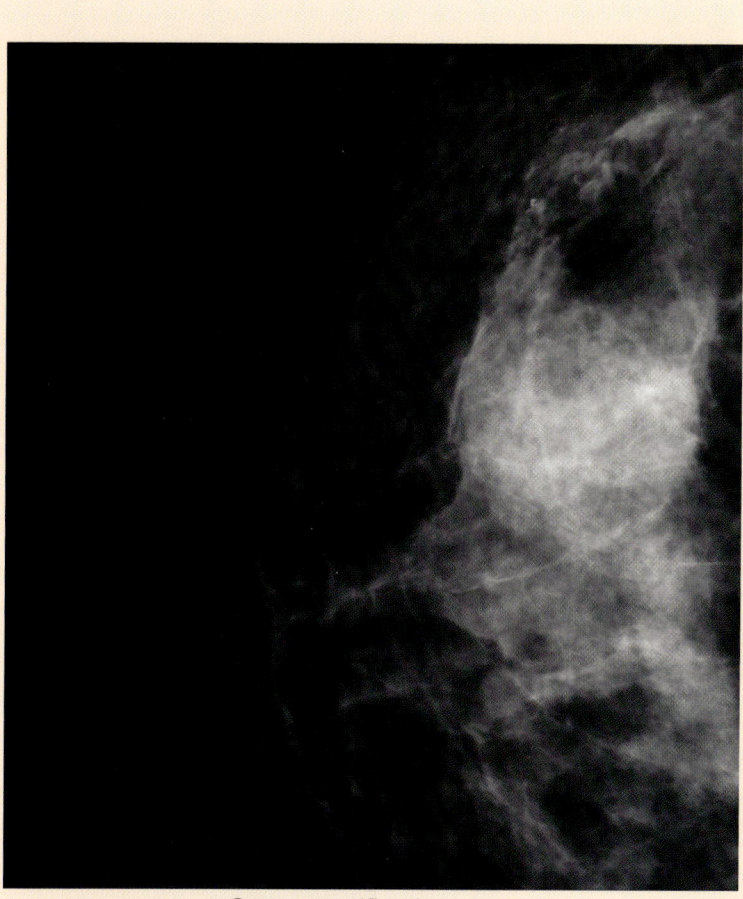

Spot magnification view

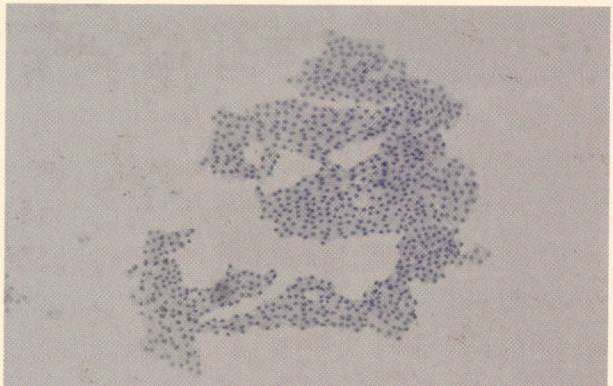

FNAC image

Key Points

In the background of heterogeneously dense breast parenchyma, outline of focal breast lesions can be partially or completely obscured, requiring further evaluation by USG/ MRI.

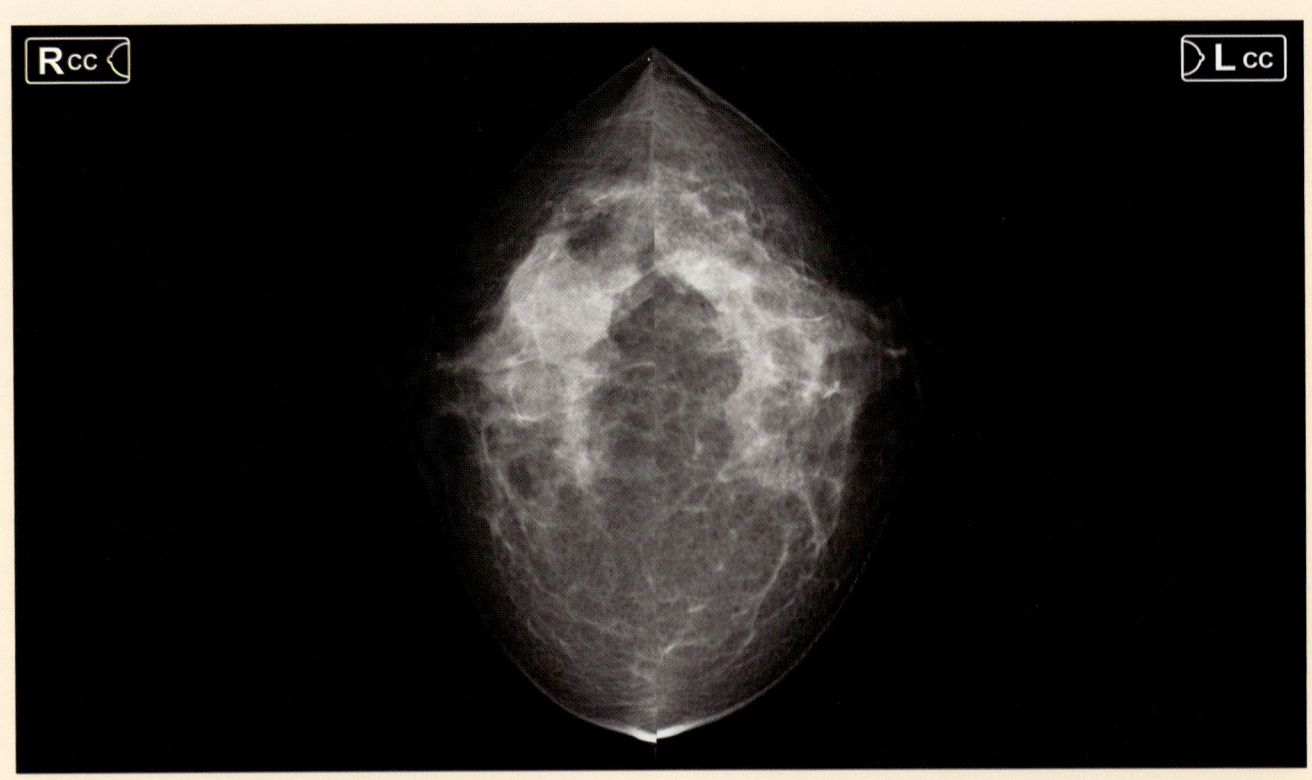

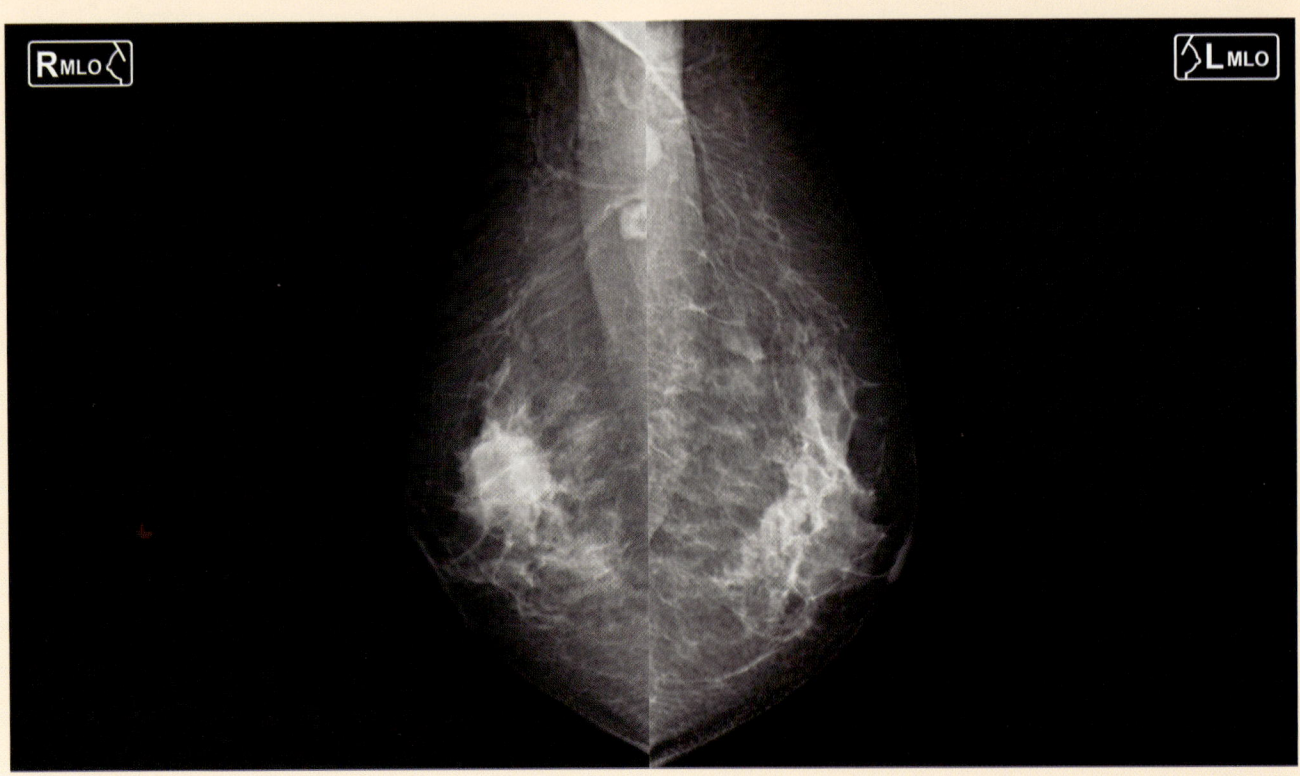

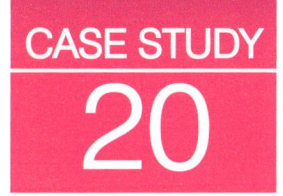
41-year-old lady with lump in left breast

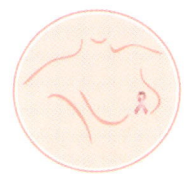

Mammography

ACR Type B density.

Left breast shows a 4.5 cm sized soft tissue lesion with smooth, geometric margins in the central quadrant. BIRADS IVa due to the size of the lesion in spite of smooth outline.

USG: Left breast shows a 4.5 cm smooth marginated hypoechoic lesion with distal acoustic enhancement in inferior quadrant. BIRADS IVa due to the size of the lesion.

USG-guided biopsy: Benign ducts and glands with foci of adenosis and stromal hyalinization. No evidence of DCIS/malignancy. Post-lumpectomy HPE showed same findings with no evidence of malignancy.

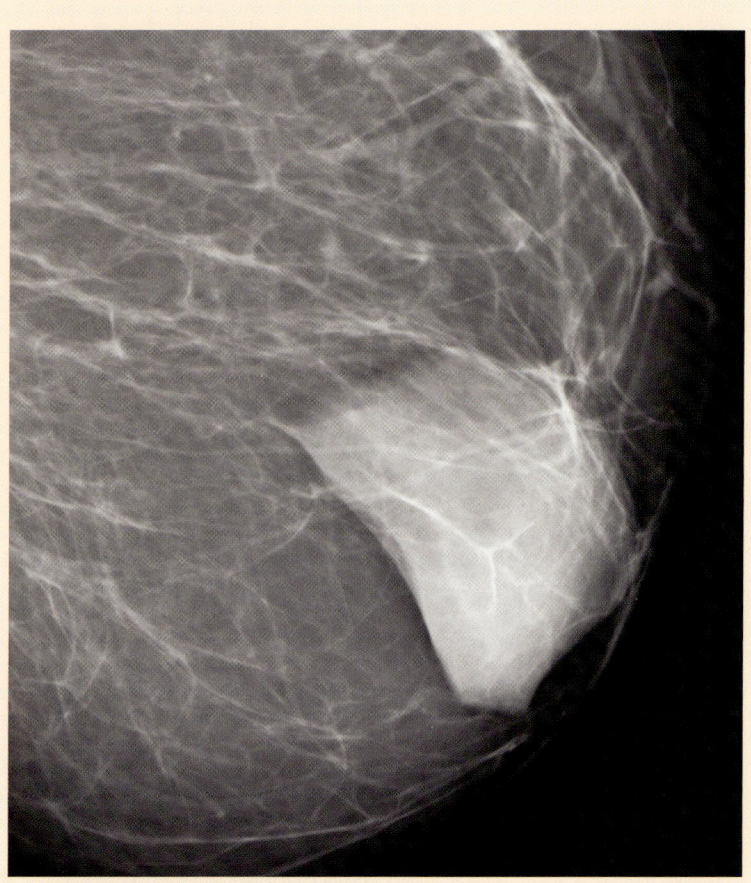

Zoomed left MLO view

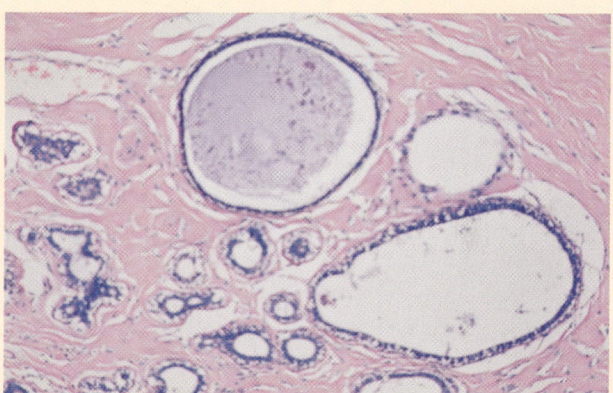

HPE image

Key Points

Malignant lesions generally do not show geometric margins. Cystic lesions, especially larger ones and soft benign lesions can be deformed and show geometric angular margins on mammography due to the compression of breast inherent in the mammography technique.

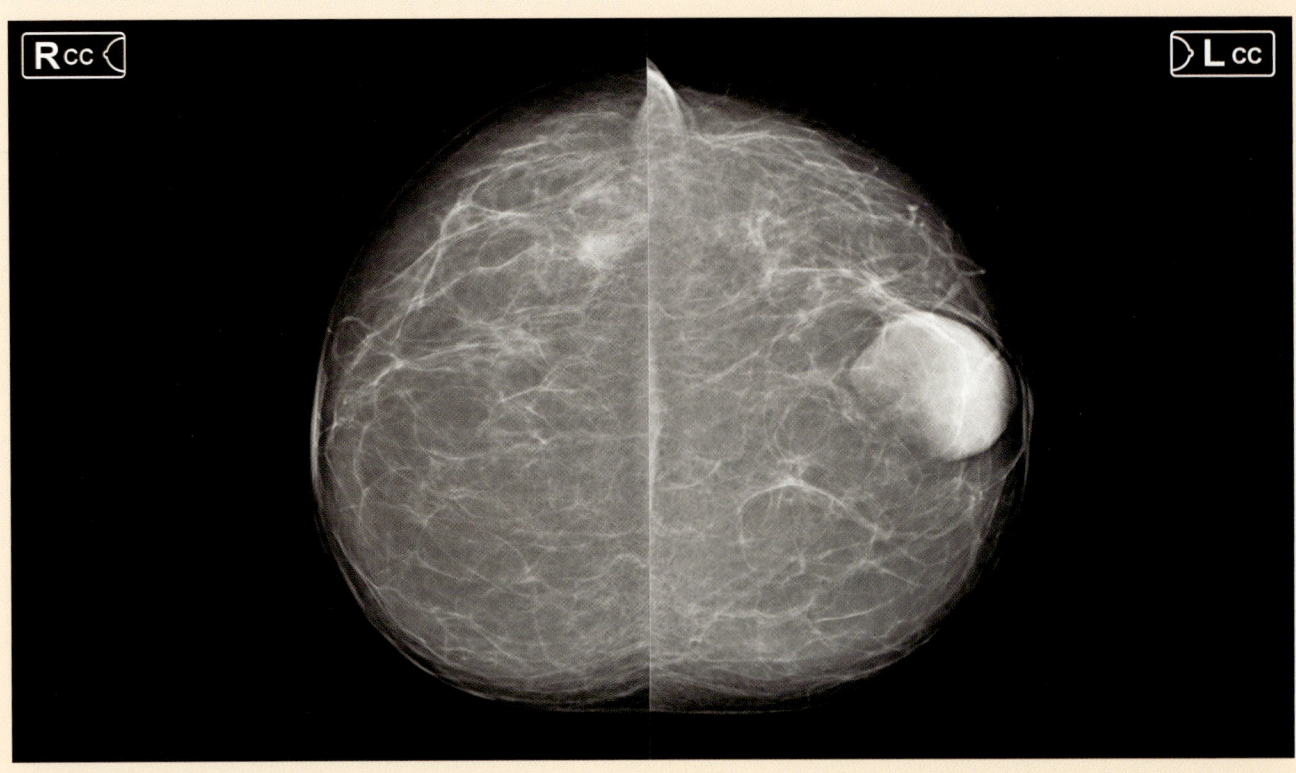

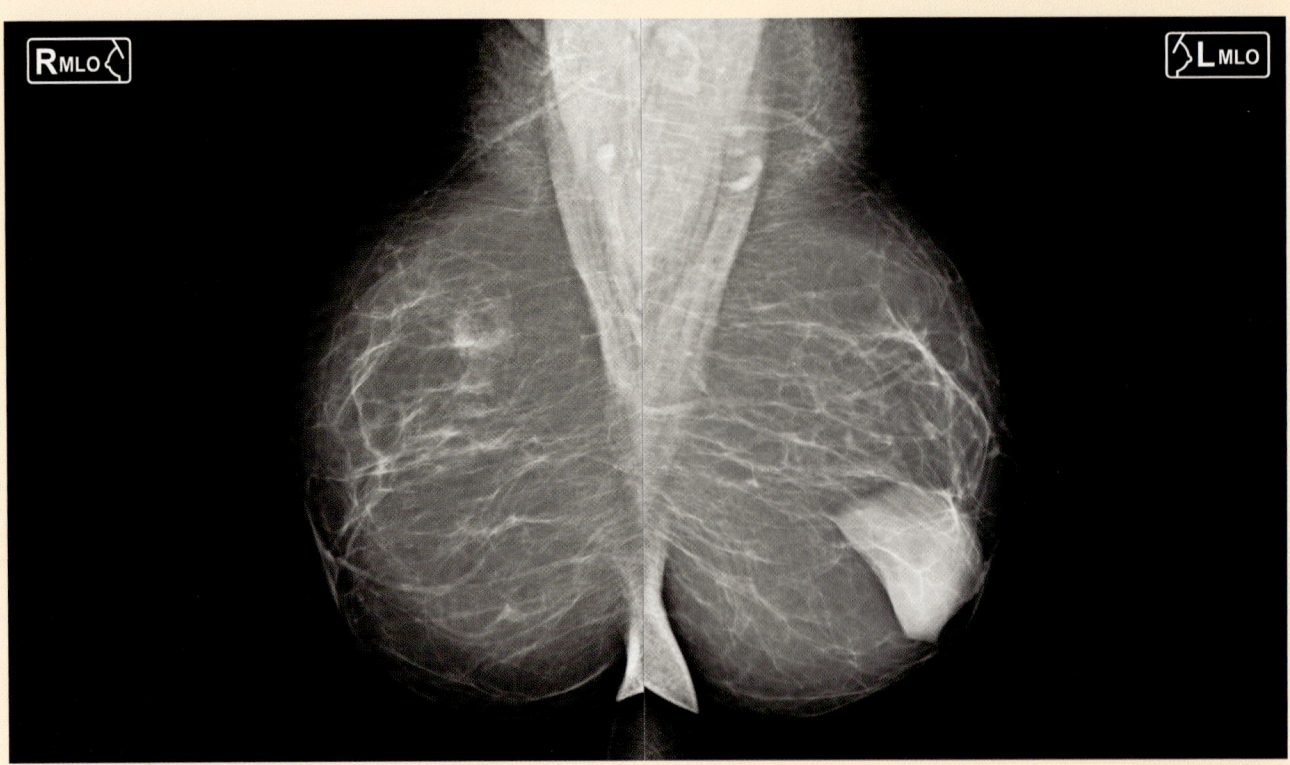

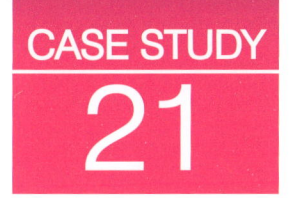
41-year-old lady with lump in left breast

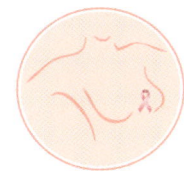

Mammography

ACR Type B density.

A smooth marginated opacity of 3 x 2.5 cm seen in upper outer quadrant of left breast. BIRADS III, suggested USG correlation, guided FNAC.

USG: Left breast shows a smooth marginated, oval hypoechoic lesion with posterior acoustic enhancement in upper outer quadrant of left breast. US - BIRADS III.

Suggested follow-up imaging after 6 months.

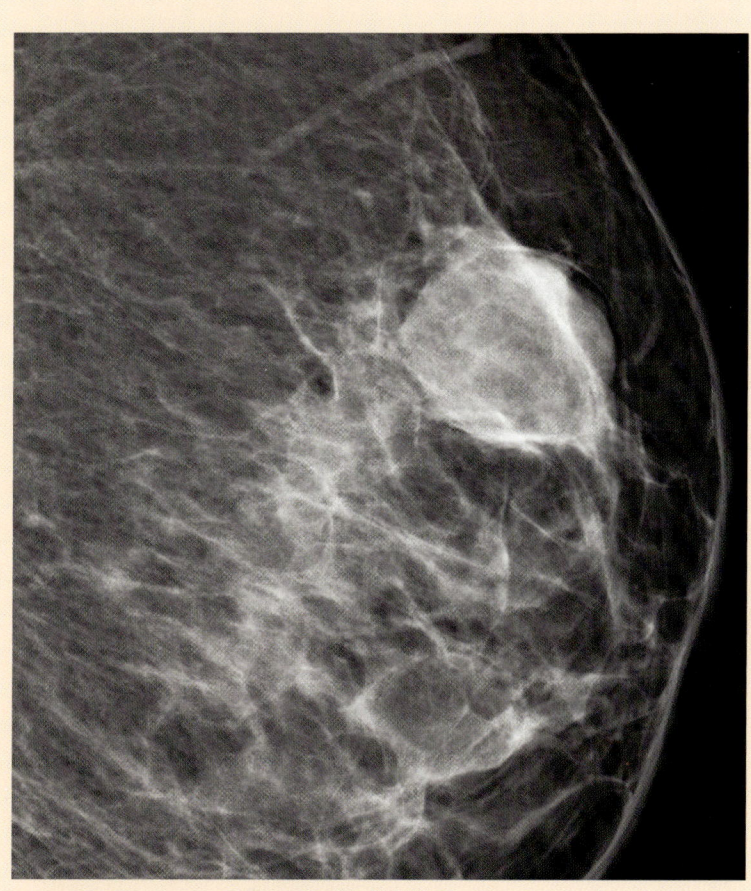

Zoomed left MLO view

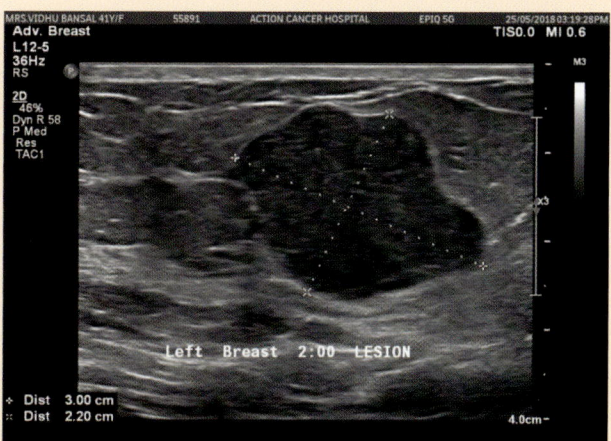

USG of left breast lesion

Key Points

If the patient refuses FNA/ HPE correlation in a solid BIRADS III lesion, short-term follow-up imaging (every 3 to 6 months) should be done for a 2-year period to establish stability of the lesion.

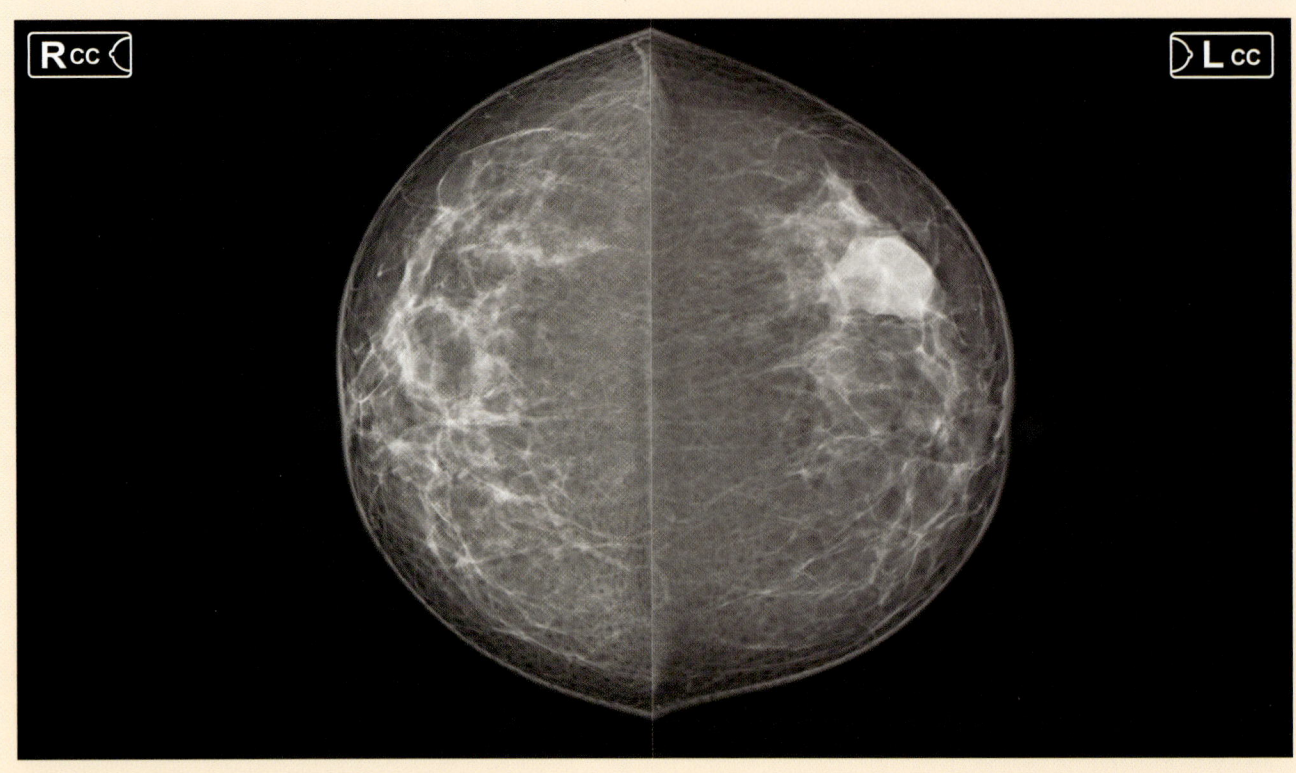

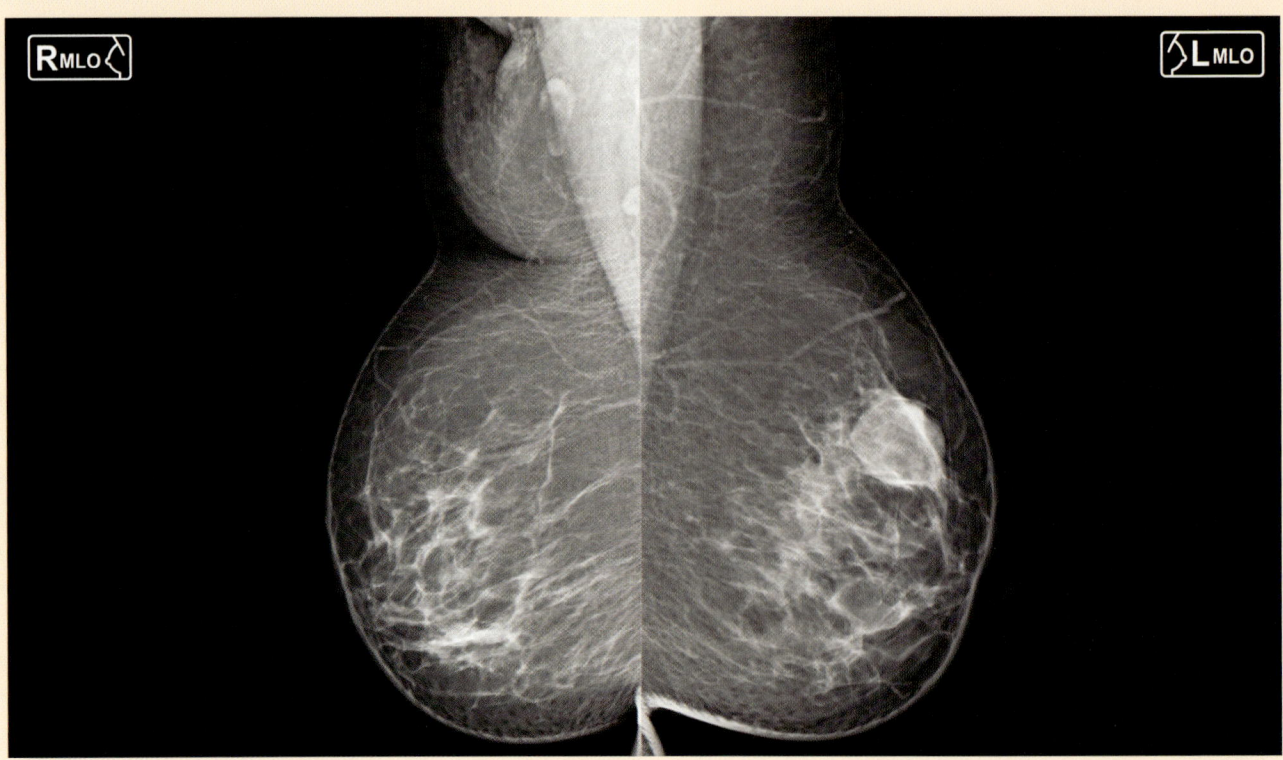

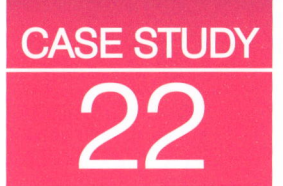
50-year-old lady with palpable lump in right breast

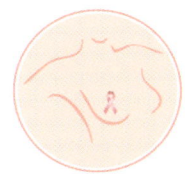

Mammography

ACR Type B density:

Right breast shows a rounded smooth marginated lesion of 2.7 cm size in upper outer quadrant with a cluster of monomorphic micro-, macro-calcifications projected over the soft tissue lesion. BIRADS 0. Further evaluation by USG suggested.

USG breast reveals a thin-walled cystic lesion of 2.8 cm size corresponding to the lesion seen on mammography.

USG-guided aspiration of cyst performed.

Fluid cytology of aspirated fluid shows features of proliferative mammary lesion with no evidence of malignancy.

Check mammogram of right breast reveals no discernible residual lesion. Clusters of benign appearing calcifications remain unchanged. Suggested follow-up mammography after 6 months for the clustered calcifications.

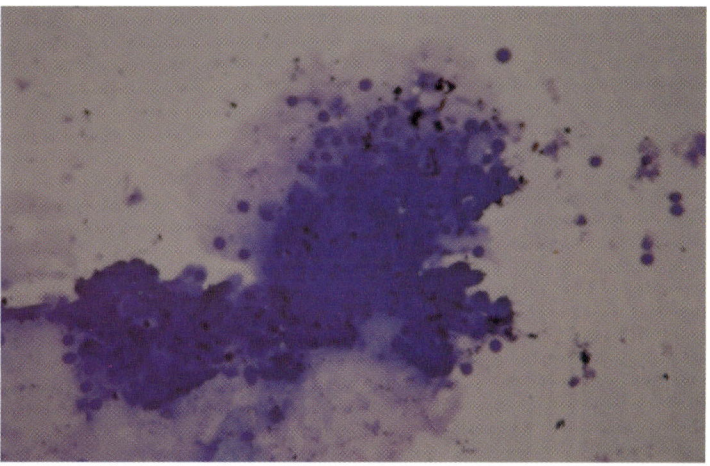

FNAC image

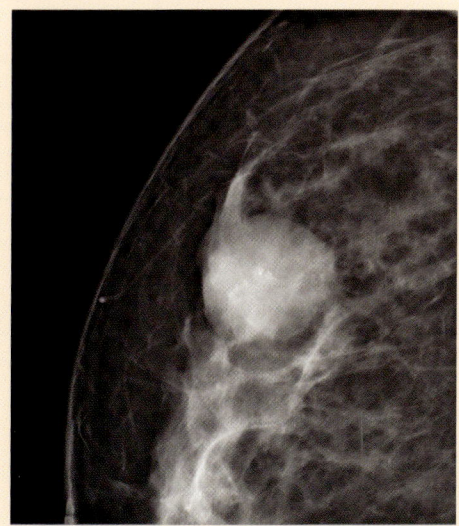

Zoomed right CC view

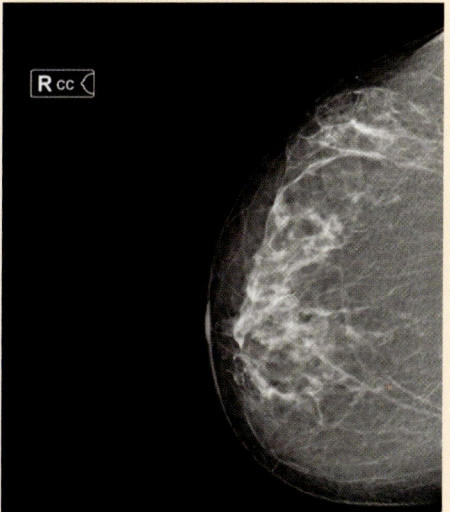

Post-aspiration check mammography image

Key Points

Cysts of concern with no discernible solid component can be aspirated to entirety under USG guidance and a check USG/mammogram performed to confirm complete resolution. If any residual abnormality remains, FNA/follow-up can be done for the same. Monomorphic clustered calcifications are generally benign and can be followed up to ensure stable appearances.

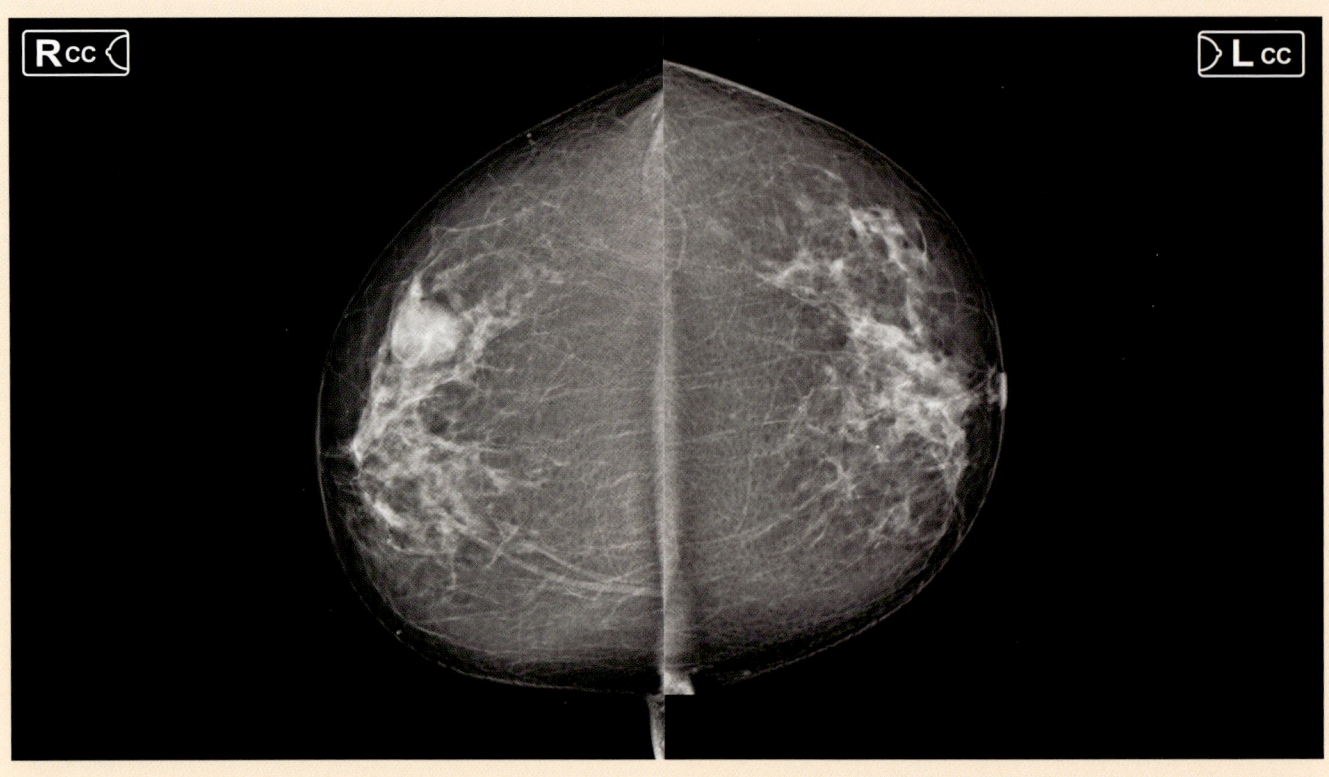

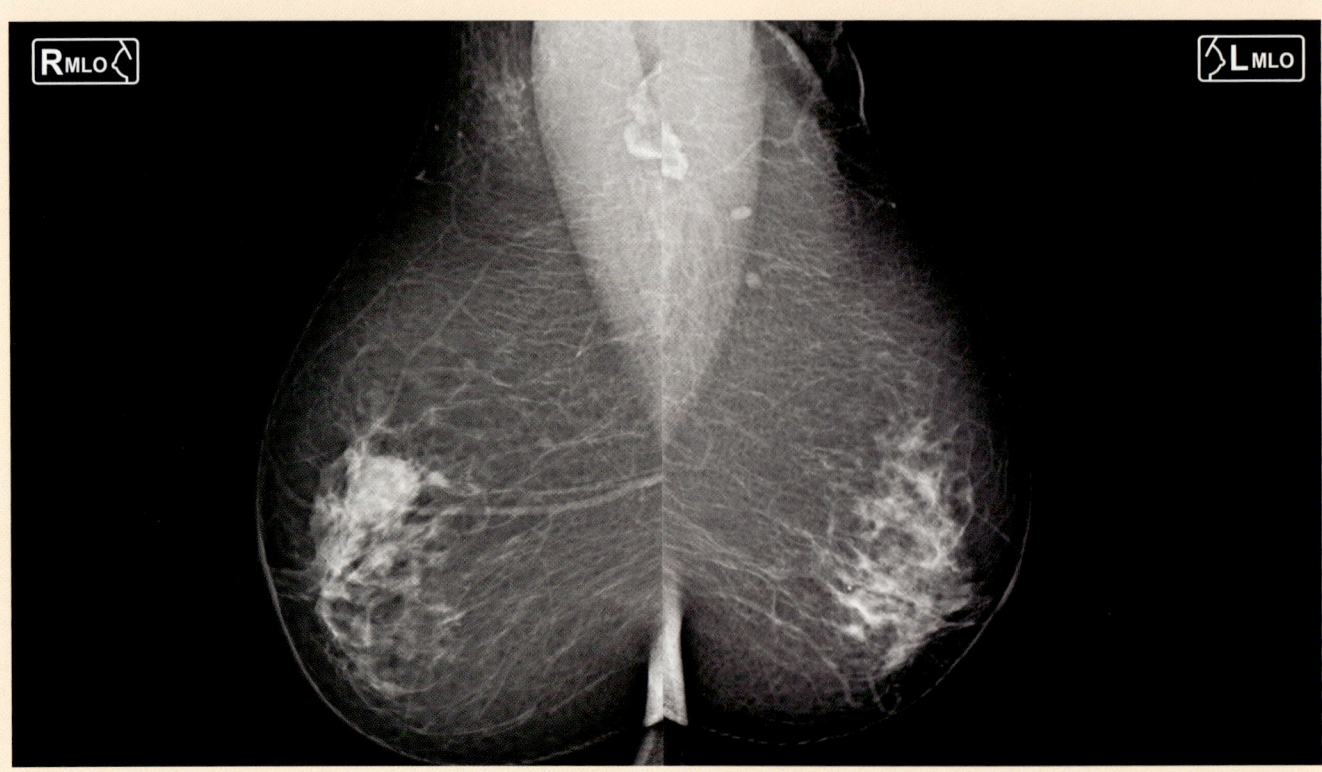

47-year-old female with bloody discharge from right nipple

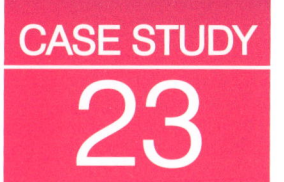
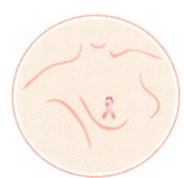

Mammography

ACR Type B density :

Right breast shows a solitary mildly dilated duct in the inner quadrant with clustered asymmetric densities in the inner quadrant along with 1.1 cm sized smooth marginated opacity in the inner quadrant. BIRADS 0 with suggested further evaluation by USG/MRI breast.

USG breast shows mildly dilated solitary duct in upper inner quadrant of right breast with no obvious intraluminal soft tissue lesion with multiple subcentimeter smooth marginated hypoechoic lesions in upper inner quadrant, further evaluation by MRI breast suggested.

Clinico-radiological meet discussion suggested offering further evaluation by MRI breast/micro-dochectomy.

Patient opted for microdochectomy for which USG-guided wire localization was done.

HPE: Ductal carcinoma *in situ* with largest focus of DCIS measuring 0.7 cm. No invasive malignancy identified.

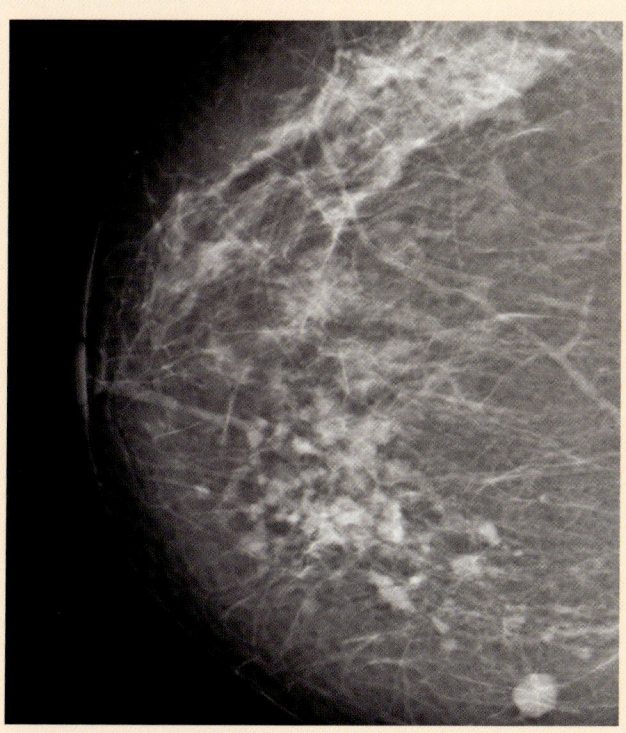

Zoomed right CC view

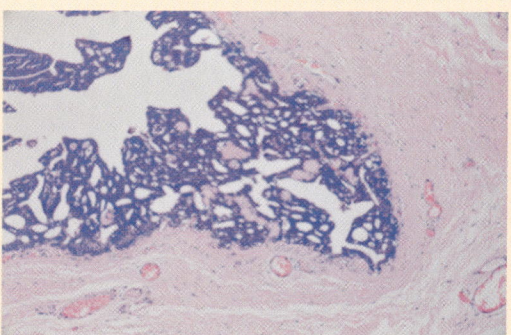

HPE image

Key Points

Solitary dilated duct and/or ductal / segmental / quadrantic soft tissue abnormalities on mammography need further evaluation by USG / MRI and any solid appearing or enhancing component would need a HPE correlation. *In situ* malignant lesions can many times appear smooth marginated on imaging and multiple smooth marginated lesions in ductal/ segmental distribution should be viewed with suspicion and evaluated further as in the case above.

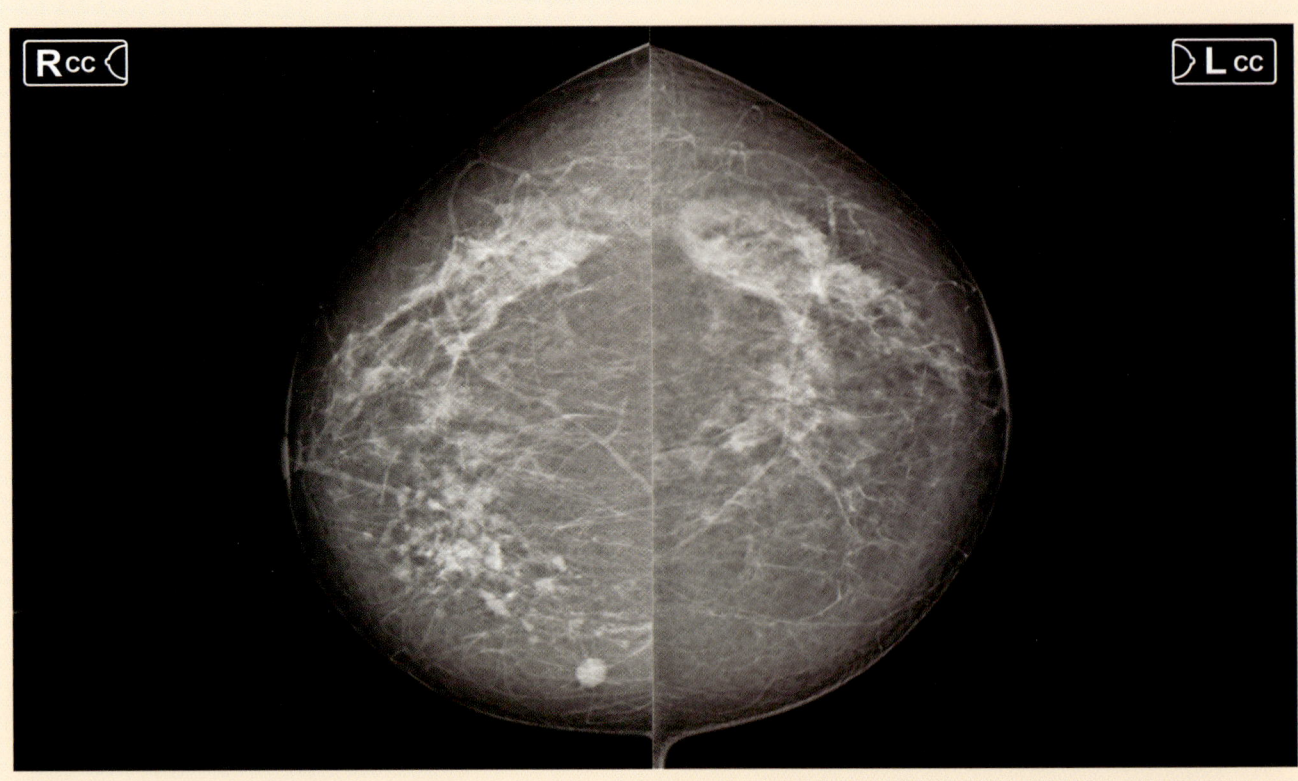

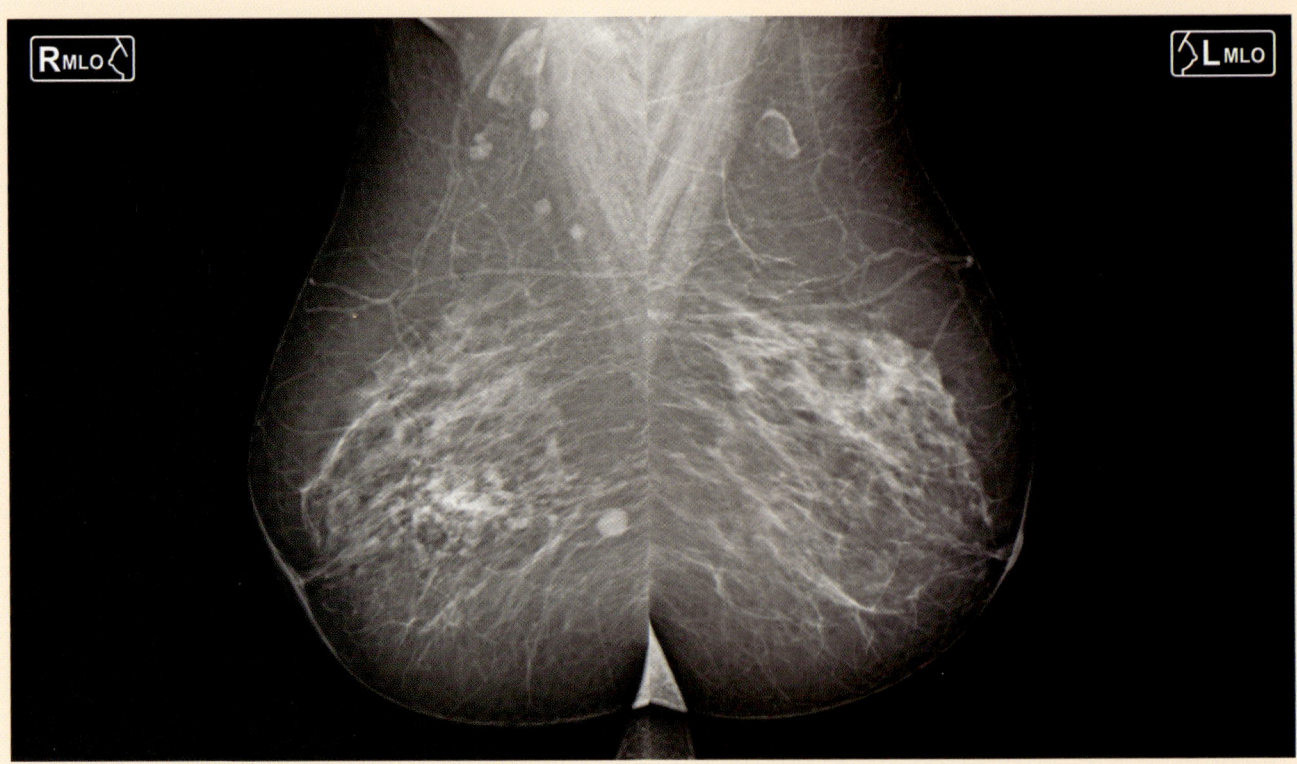

54-year-old female presenting with a lump in left breast

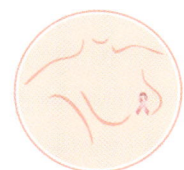

Mammography

ACR Type A density.

Left breast shows a rounded soft tissue lesion in the inferomedial quadrant. The lesion shows irregular outline with mild architectural distortion around the lesion.

BIRADS V

Left MRM HPE: Invasive mammary carcinoma.

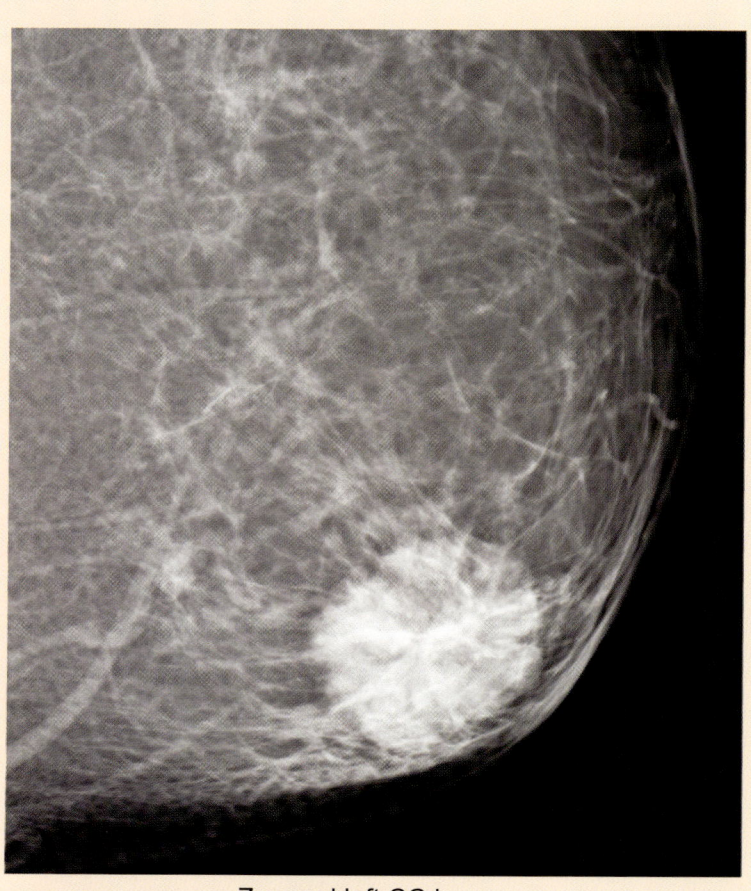

Zoomed left CC image

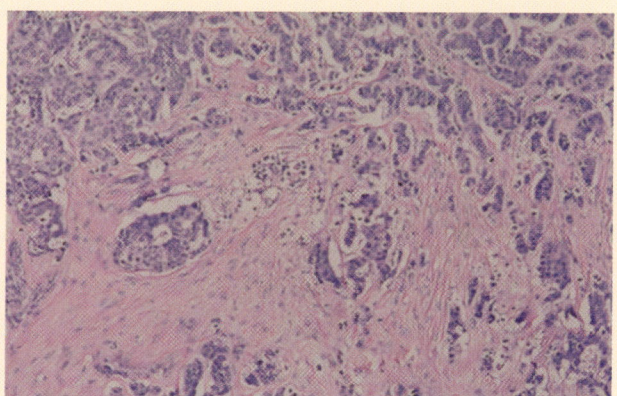

MRM HPE image

Key Points

Rounded high density mass with irregular outline and architectural distortion is a classical appearance of malignant lesion.

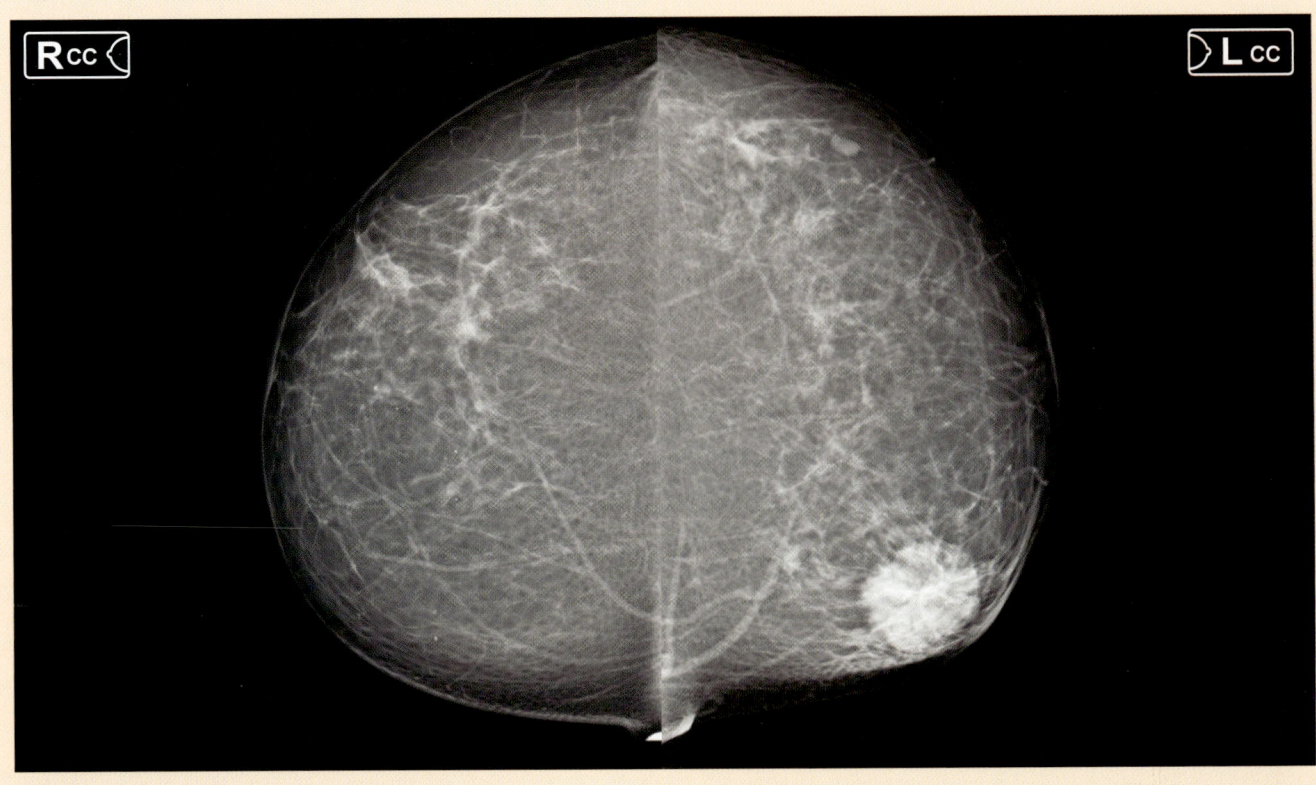

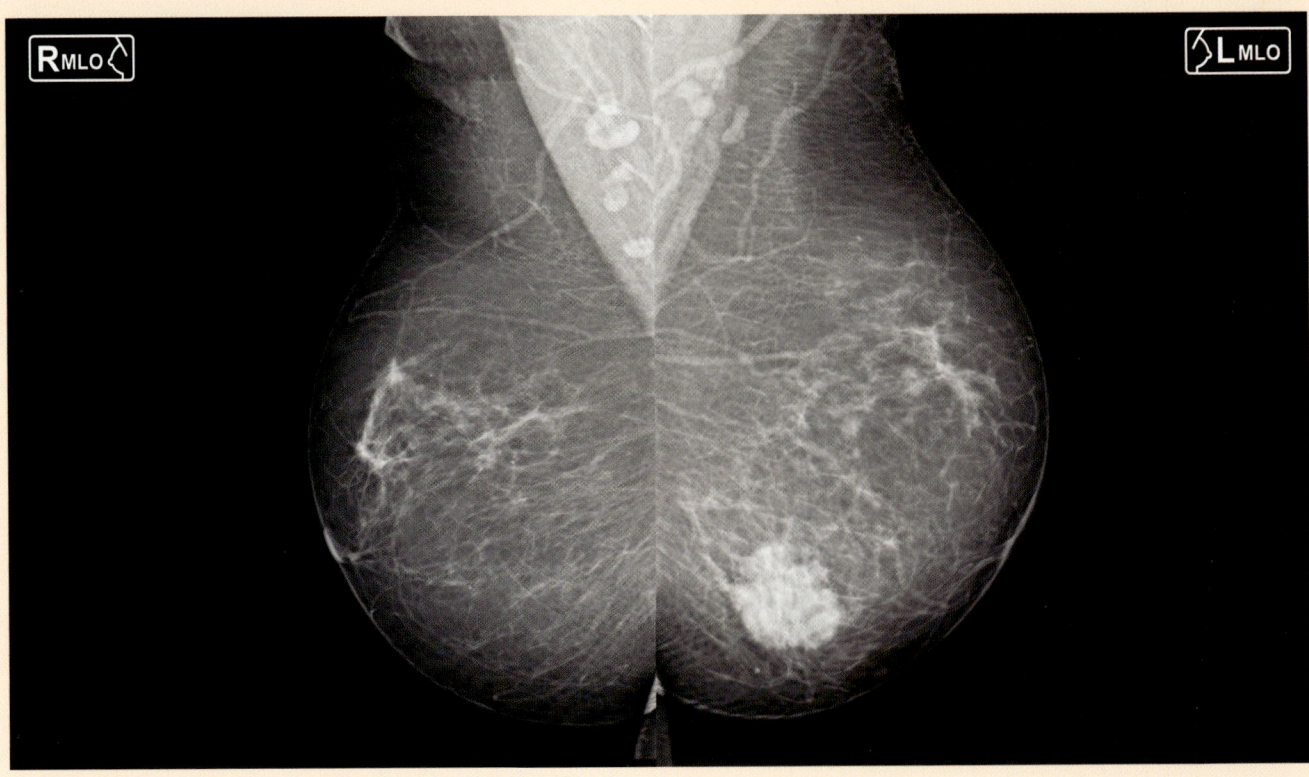

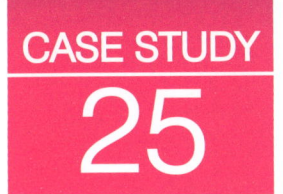
69-year-old lady with lump in right breast

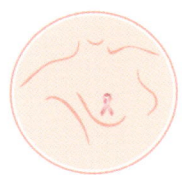

Mammography

ACR Type A density.

Rounded soft tissue lesion in upper quadrant of right breast with a tiny marginal macrocalcification. The margin of lesion is partially obscured by adjacent breast parenchyma. Spot magnification shows irregular outline of a portion with smooth margins in the rest of the lesion. No associated architectural distortion. BIRADS IVc. Suggested FNA / Bx correlation.

USG-guided FNAC shows atypical cells in papillary projection with scant to moderate cytoplasm, round nucleus overall features positive for malignancy.

MRM HPE suggestive of papillary carcinoma.

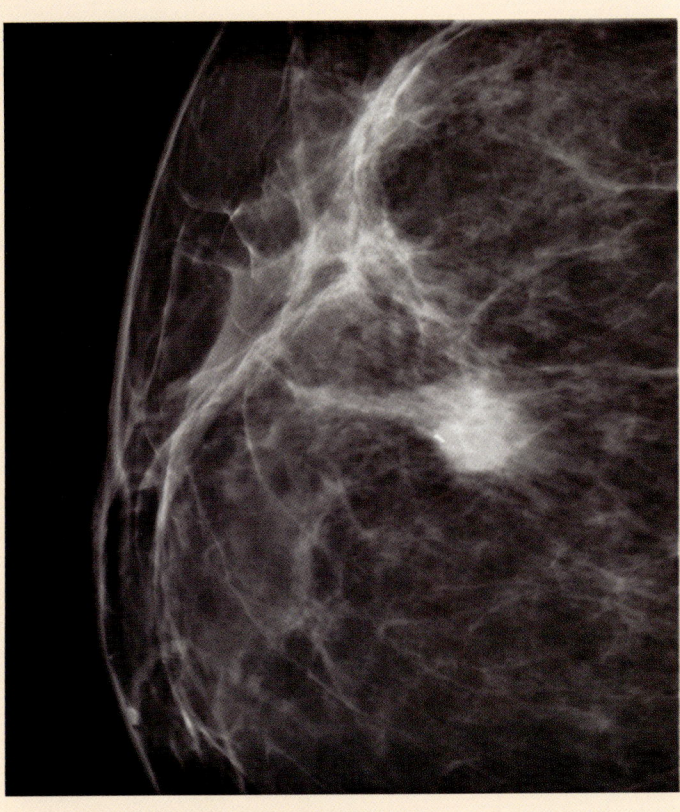

Zoomed right CC view

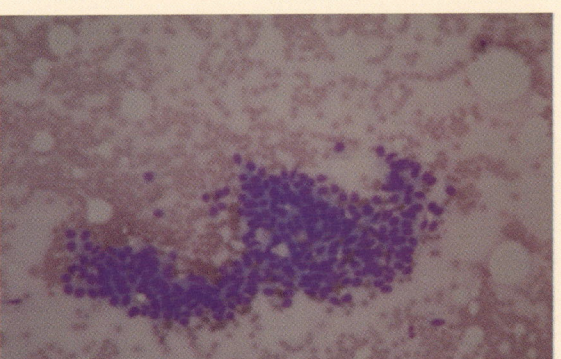

MRM HPE image

Key Points

It is important to evaluate the entire margin of any lesion. Focal irregularity in a lesion is as suspicious as diffusely irregular margin in a lesion. If a portion of the lesion's margin is obscured by overlapping breast glandular shadows, further evaluation by tomosynthesis or spot magnification view must be undertaken.

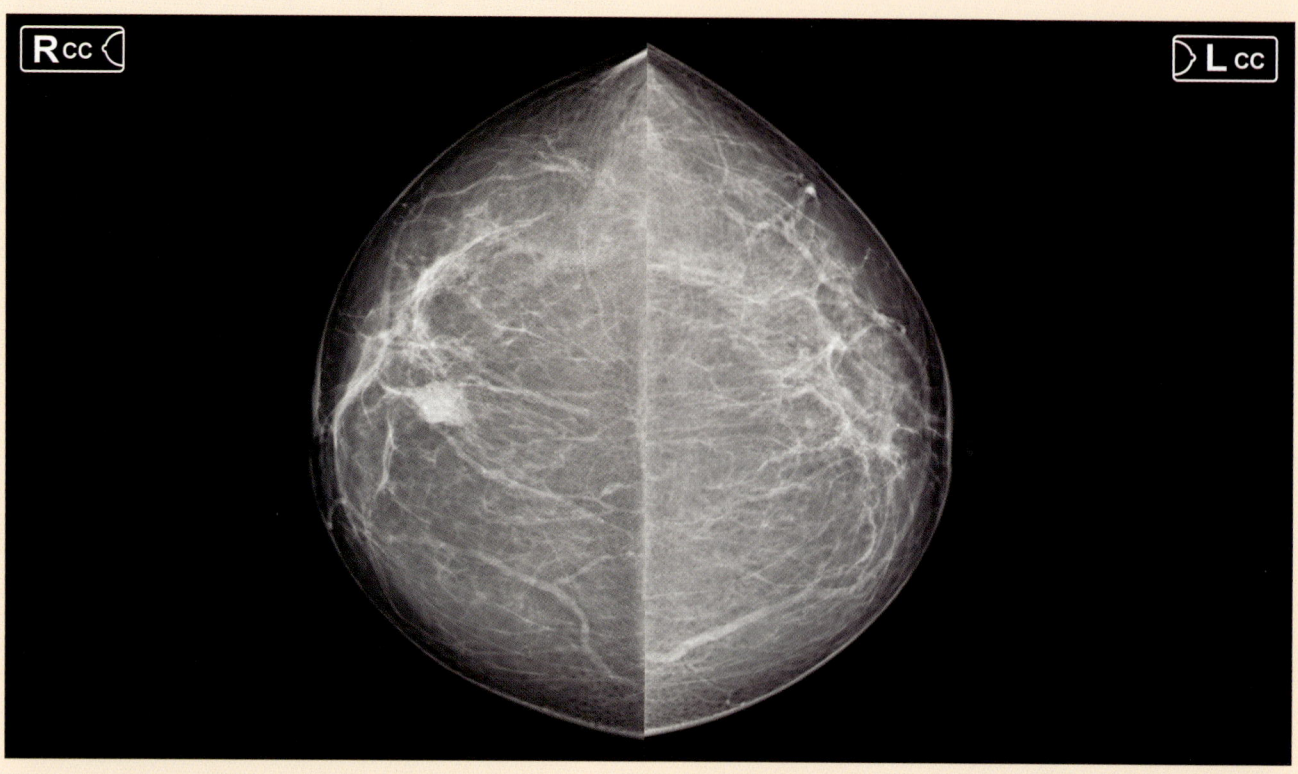

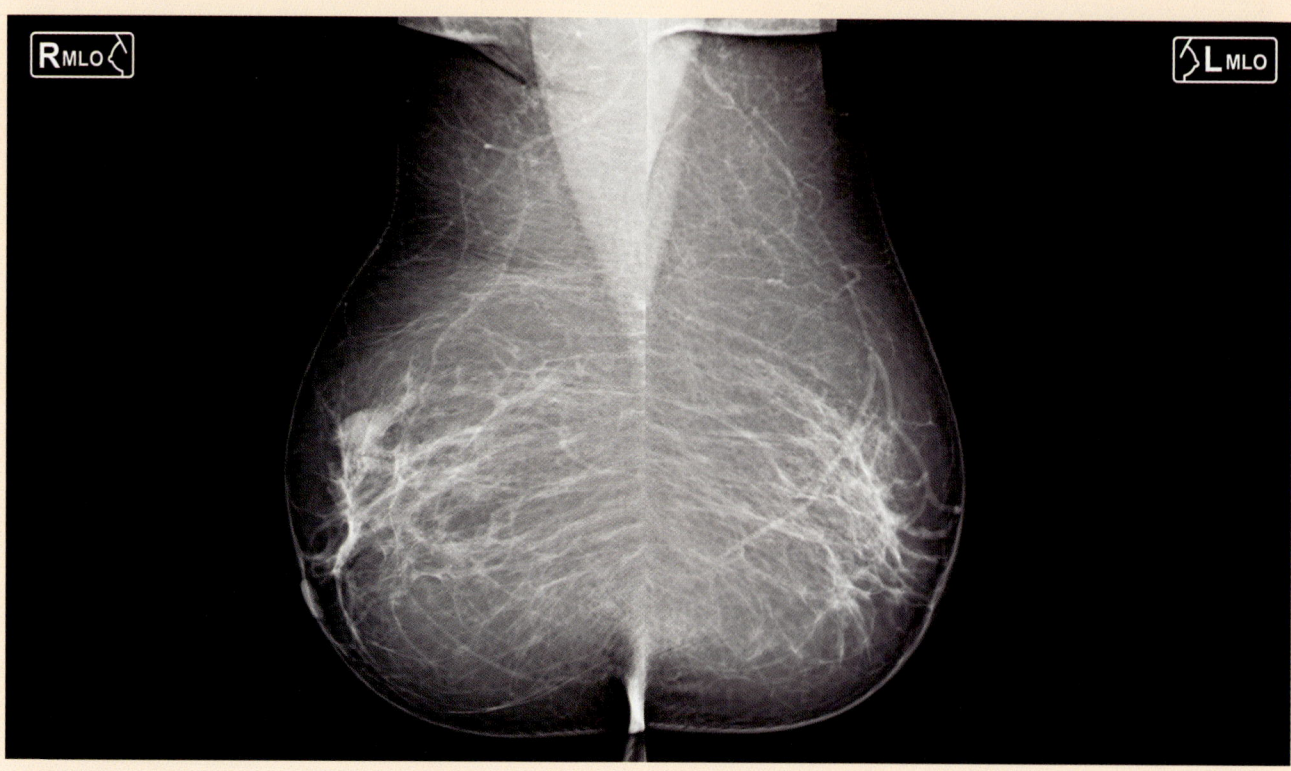

34-year-old lady presented with lump in right axilla for a few months

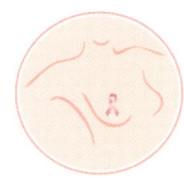

Mammography

ACR Type C density.

Smooth marginated soft tissue lesion of 2.8 cm size in right axilla. BIRADS III. Suggested USG breast correlation.

USG breast: Smooth marginated hypoechoic lesion in right axilla. BIRADS III. Follow-up imaging after 6 months/HPE correlation.

USG-guided FNAC: C3 code, suggested biopsy.

USG-guided biopsy: Proliferative breast lesion. No evidence of malignancy.

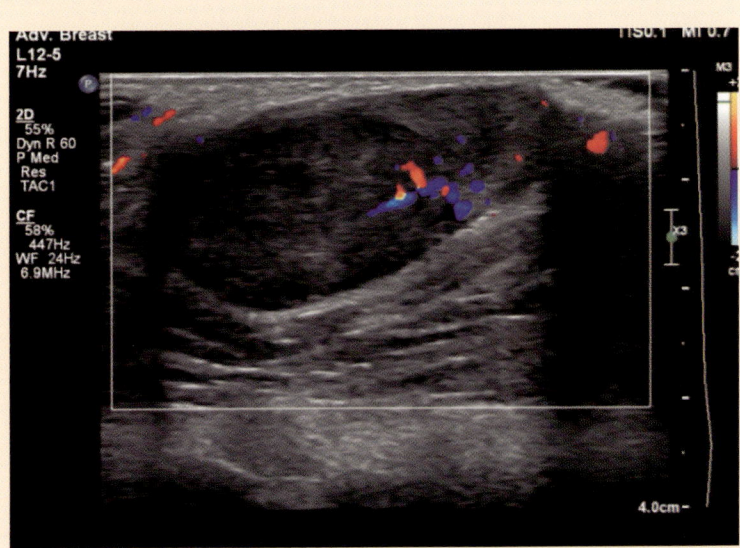

USG-Doppler image of right axillary lesion

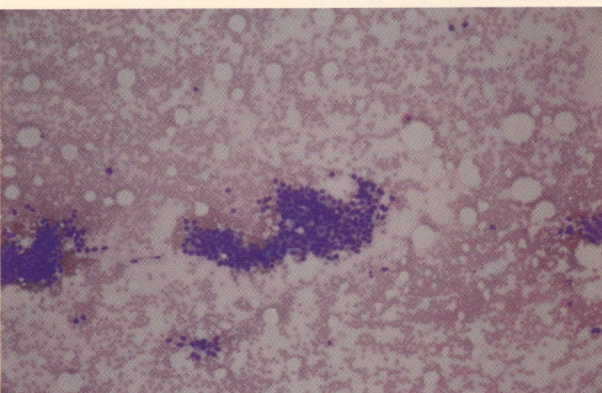

FNAC image

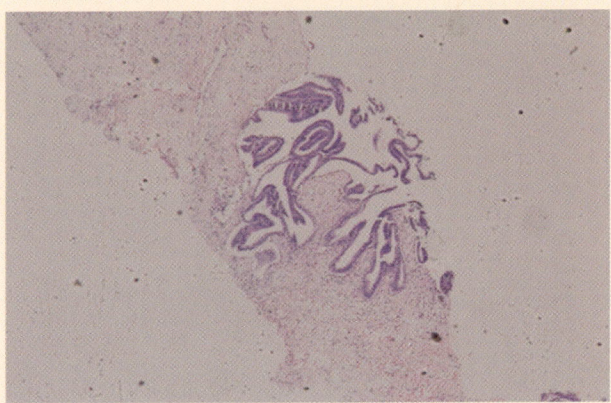

HPE image

Key Points

Focal lesions in the axillary tail of the breast may be mistaken for enlarged nodes. Absence of any central lucency and presence of fibroglandular tissue around the lesion suggests possibility of a breast parenchymal lesion. Axillary tail lesions are many times not seen on CC view as in this case. Additionally, an oval lesion may appear rounded in a single view due to projection, as in this case.

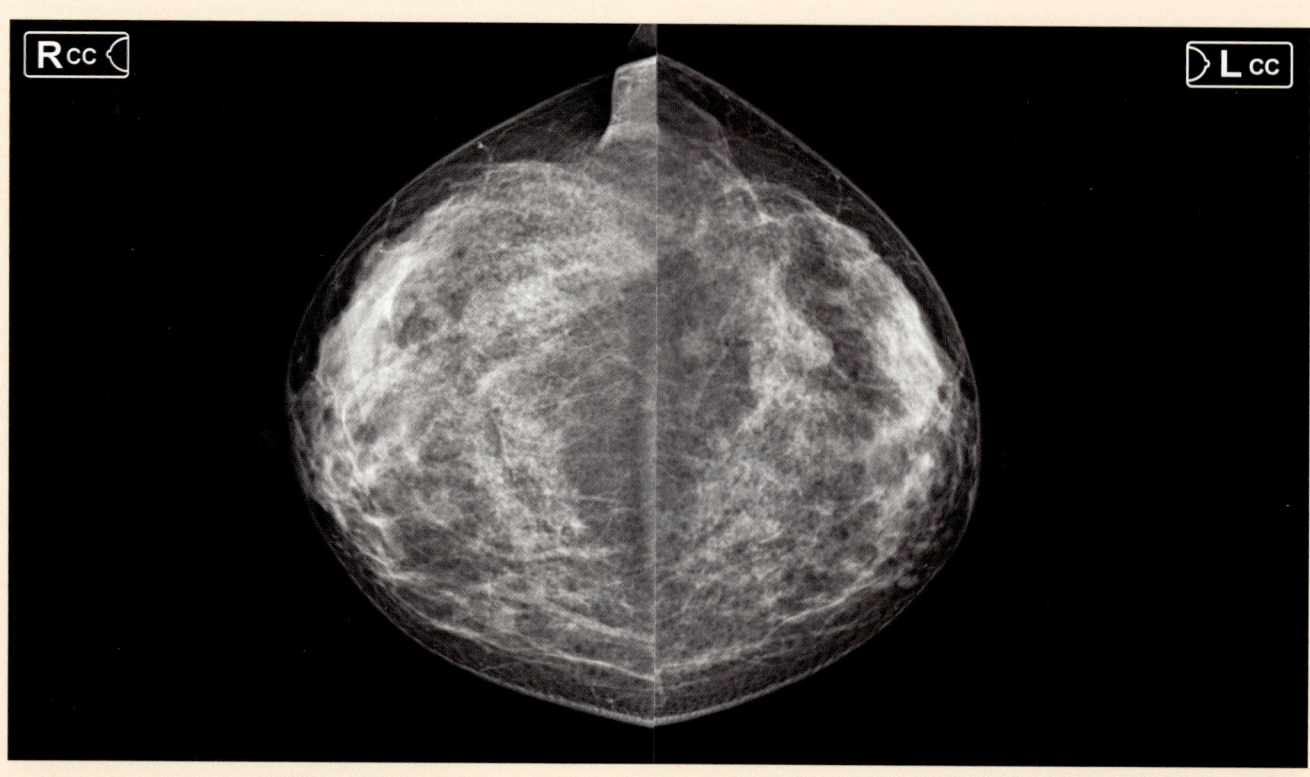

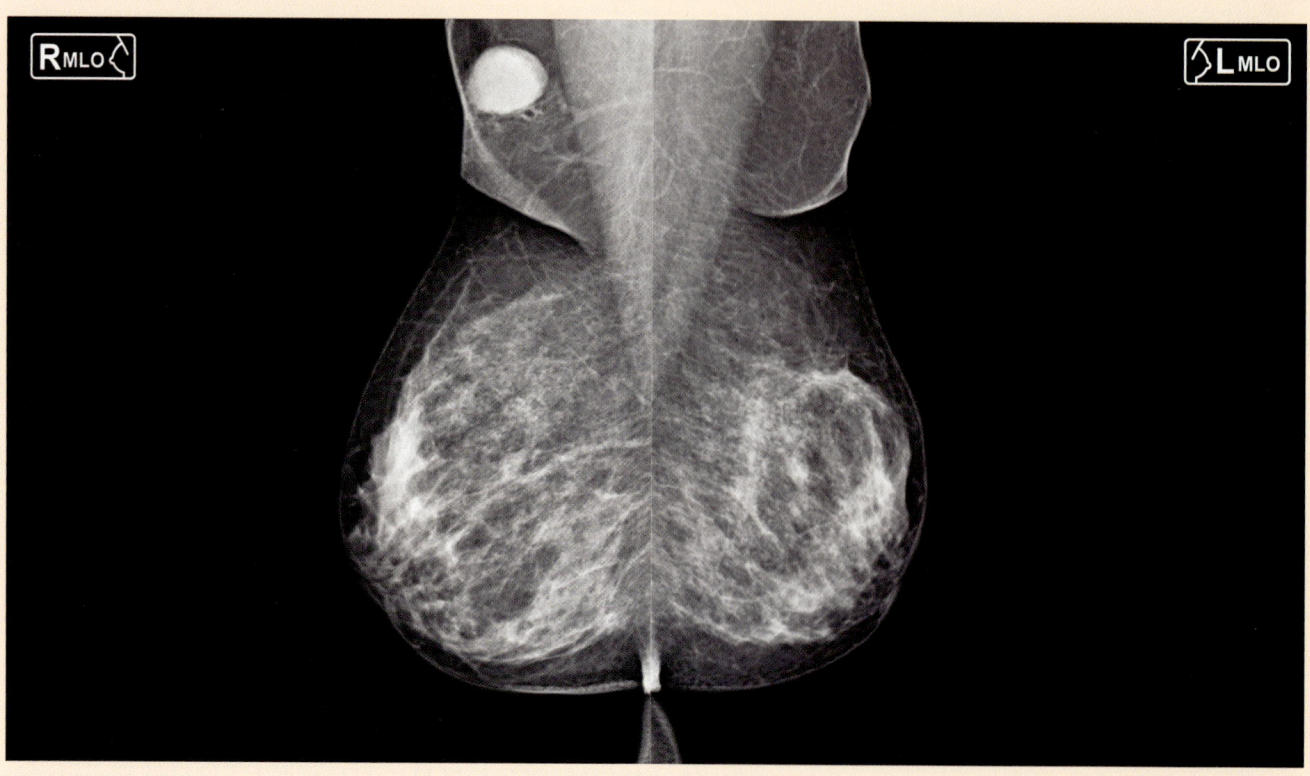

36-year-old lady presenting with lump in both breasts

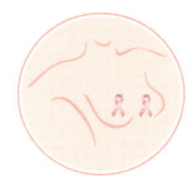

Mammography

ACR Type B density.

Multiple smooth marginated lesions in left breast, one of them showing coarse marginal calcification. A smaller smooth marginated soft tissue lesion in upper outer quadrant of right breast. BIRADS III. Suggested USG correlation and follow-up/HPE correlation.

USG breast shows smooth marginated oval hypo-echoic lesions in both breasts.

Patient opted for bilateral lumpectomy instead of follow-up.

HPE : Bilateral breast fibroadenoma.

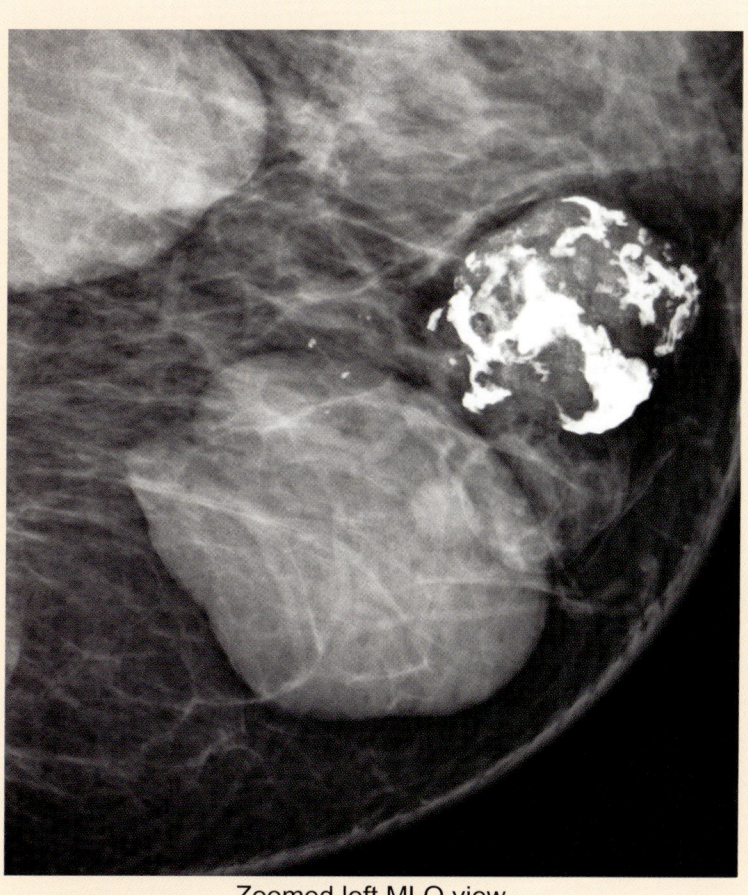

Zoomed left MLO view

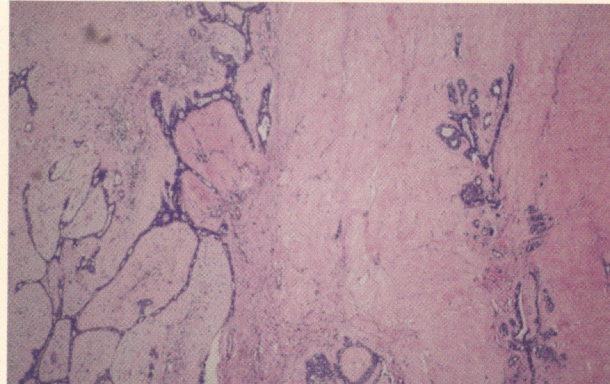

HPE soft tissue lesion

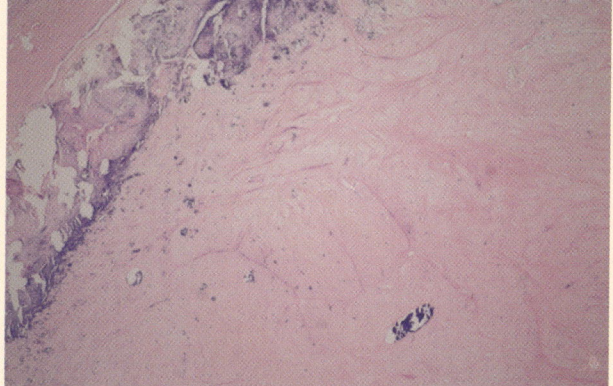

HPE calcific lesion

Key Points

In the setting of multiple lesions, all lesions need to evaluated for morphological features. All solid appearing oval, smooth marginated lesions, though likely benign, should either be followed on imaging at 3 to 6 months or undergo image guided / excision biopsy correlation.

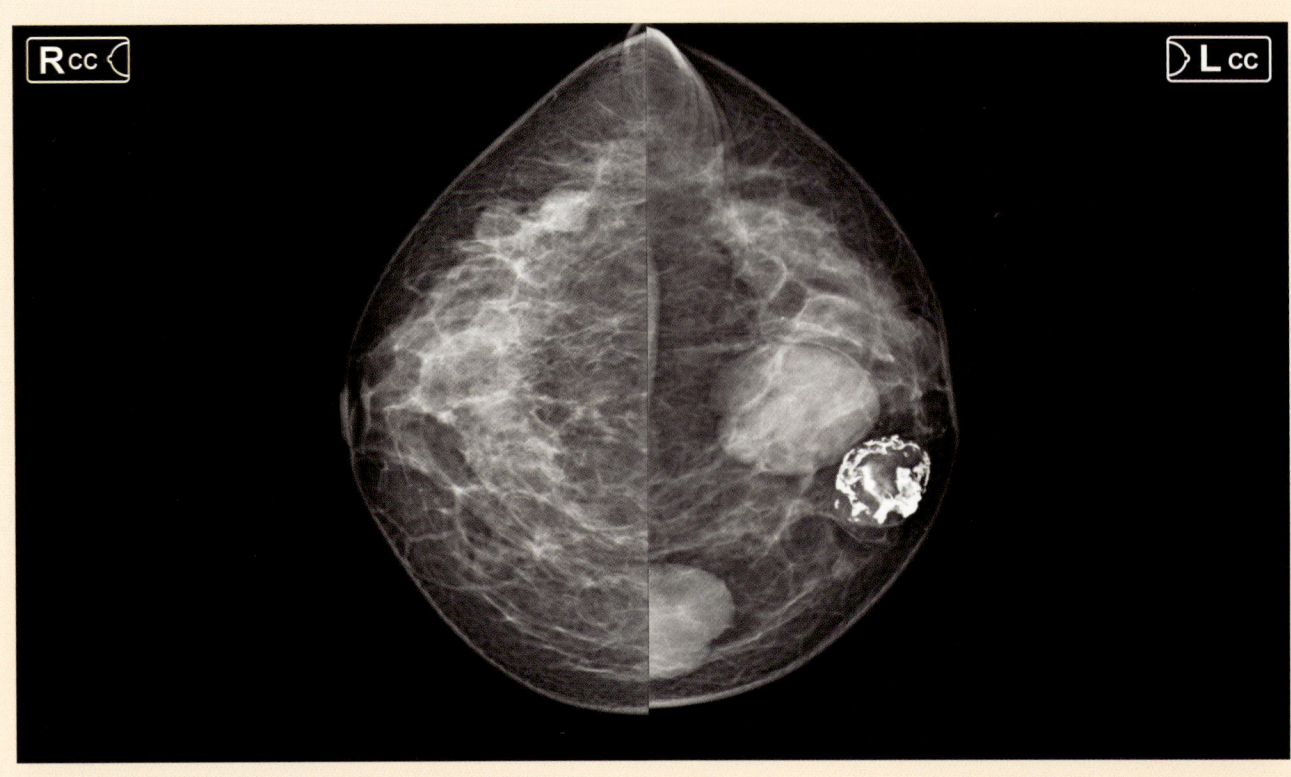

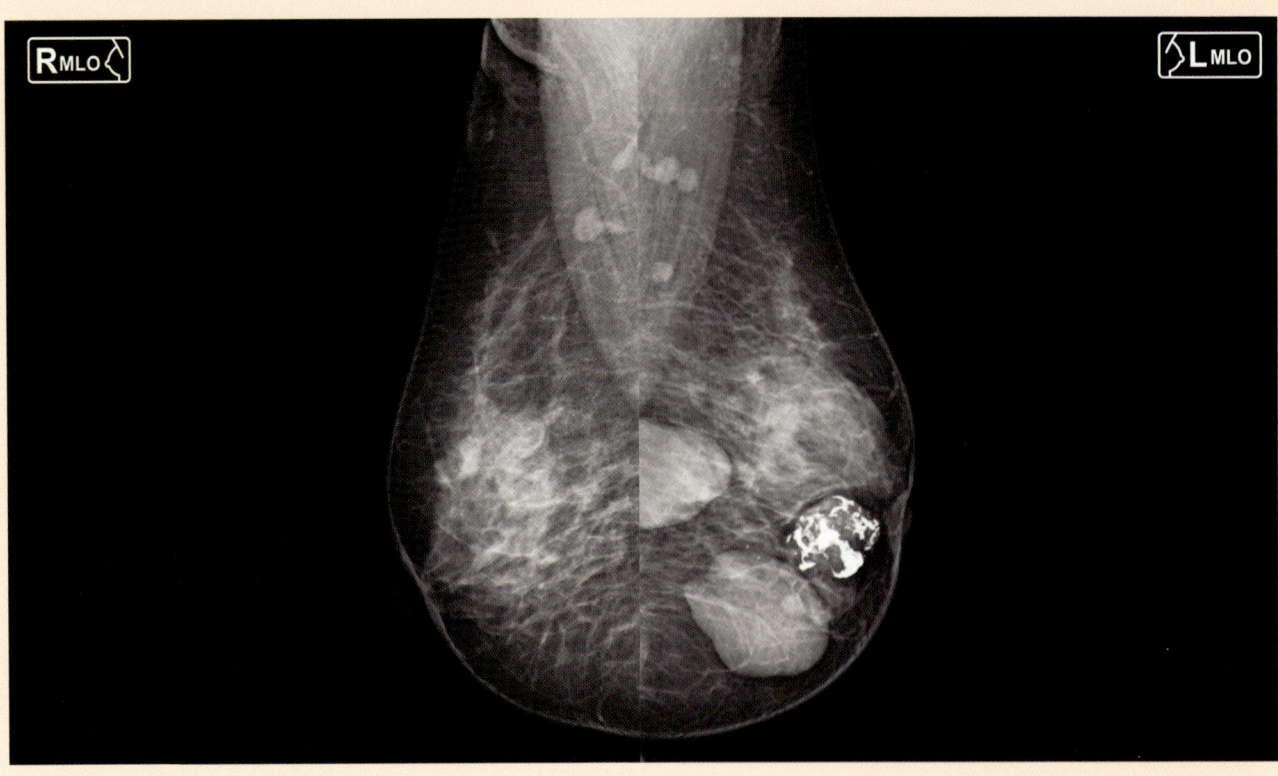

45-year-old lady presenting with left breast lumps

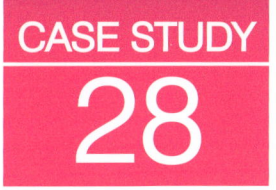
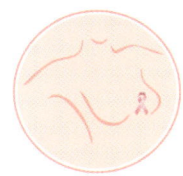

Mammography

ACR Type B density.

Asymmetric density in upper central quadrant of left breast. Additional small smooth marginated soft tissue opacity in the upper outer quadrant with Internal pleomorphic microcalcifications. Spot magnification view taken for the asymmetric density in central quadrant shows a soft tissue mass lesion with irregular margins in the central quadrant (BIRADS V) with smooth marginated lesion in outer quadrant showing internal pleomorphic microcalcifications (BIRADS V).

USG-guided FNAC from the central quadrant lesion shows features suspicious of malignancy (C4).

USG-guided FNAC from outer quadrant lesion suggested cystic papillary neoplasm suspicious for malignancy.

Patient underwent MRM.

HPE of surgical specimen revealed both breast lesions to be invasive mammary carcinoma of no special type with foci of DCIS.

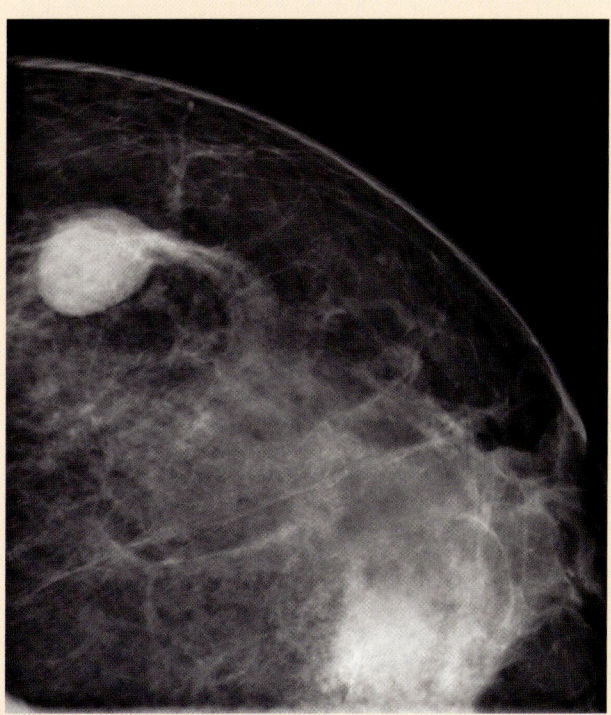

Zoomed view of left breast outer quadrant

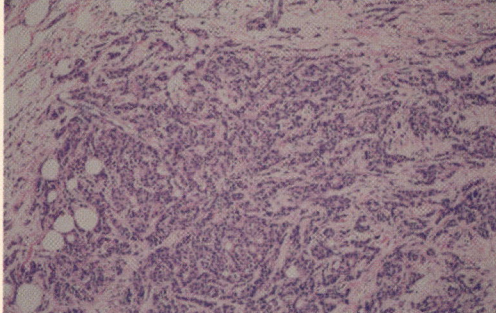

Central quadrant lesion: Invasive ductal carcinoma

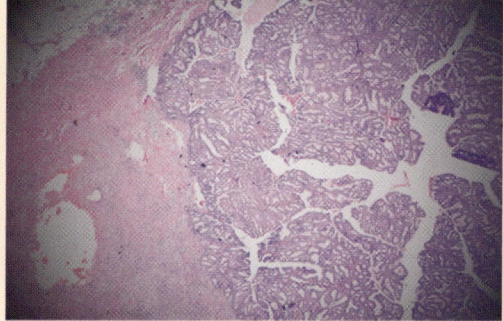

Outer quadrant lesion: Solid papillary carcinoma

Key Points

Smooth marginated lesions can be malignant. Associated findings of internal microcalcifications and presence of another focal lesion of BIRADS V morphology in this case were the reasons for categorizing the smooth marginated lesion of outer quadrant to be BIRADS V.

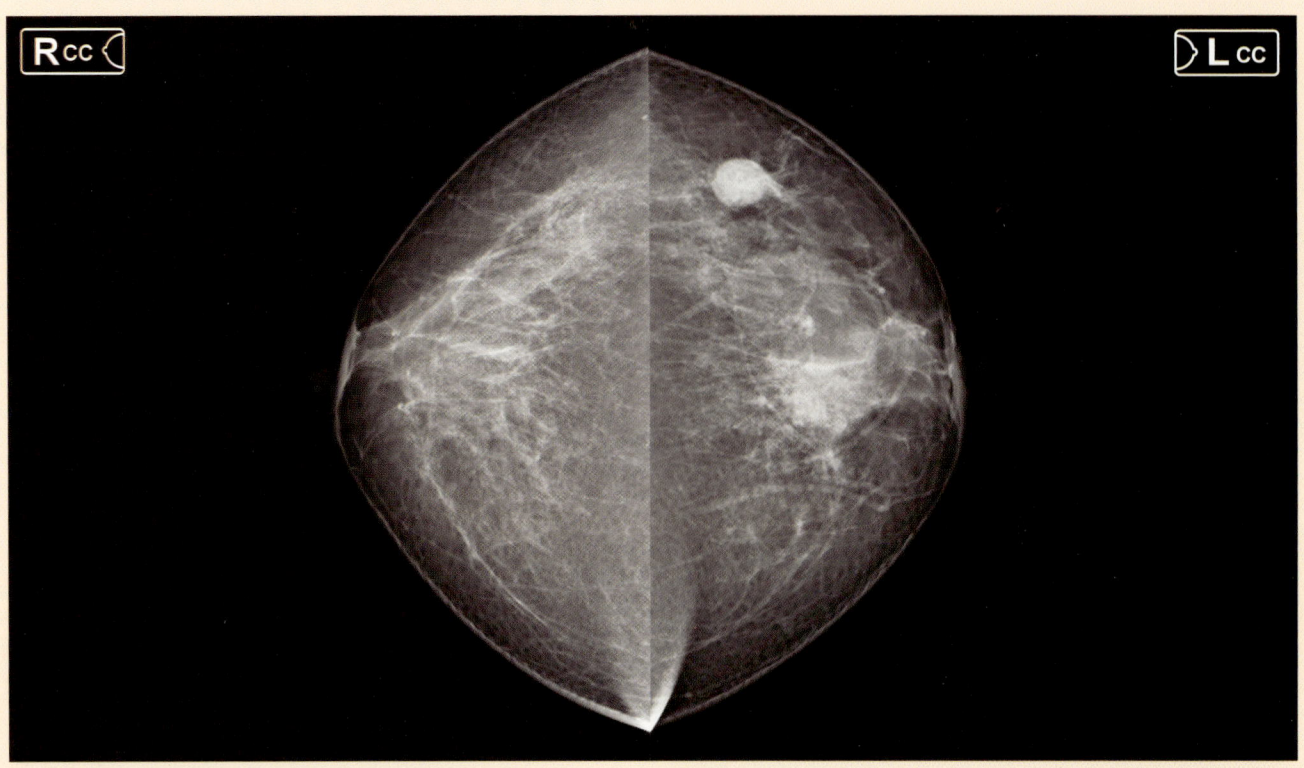

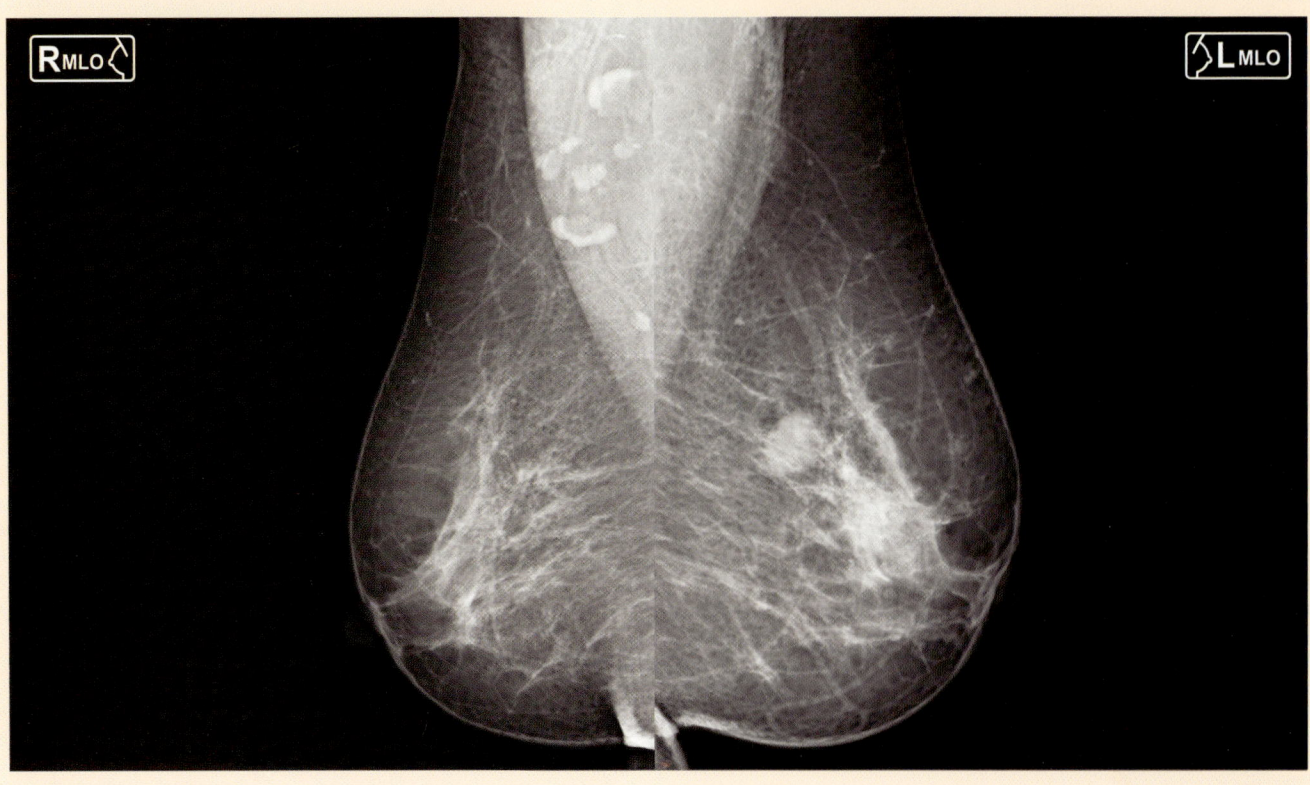

41-year-old lady presenting with right breast lump

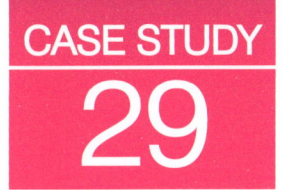
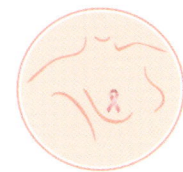

Mammography

ACR type A density.

Oval soft tissue lesion of size 4.7 x 3 cm in upper-outer quartant of right breast. The lesion shows irregularity of outline in greater then one-third of its circumference with smooth rest of margins. No significant architectural distorion microcalcifications.

BIRADS V. Suggested USG-guided biopsy.

USG showed findings similar to mammography with USG-guided biopsy showing intraductal invasive carcinoma.

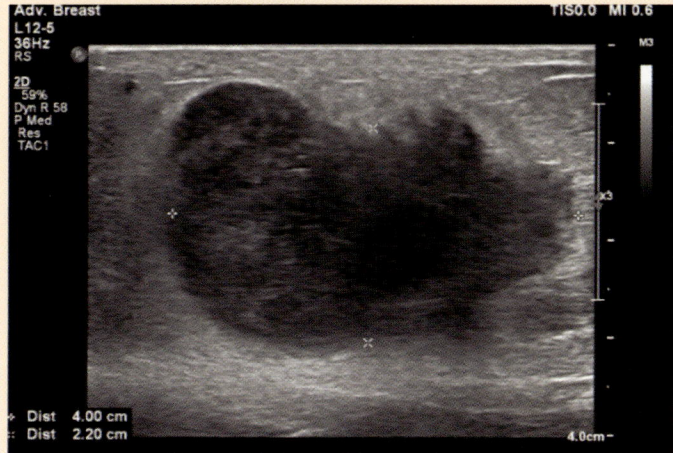

USG of right breast lesion

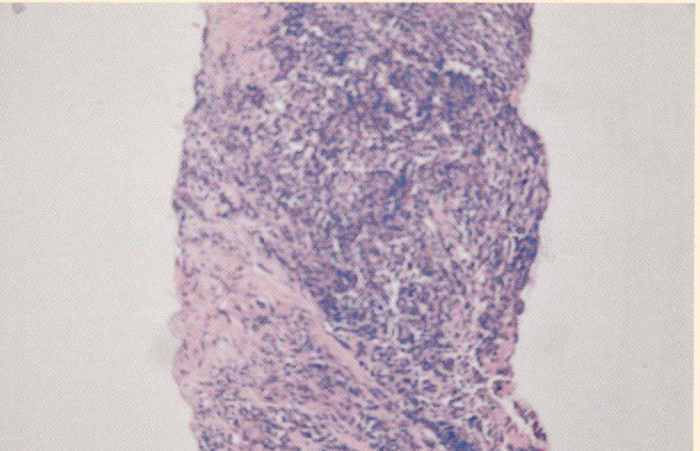

HPE image

Key Points

Focal irregularity of outline in an otherwise smooth marginated lesion is highly suspicious of underlying malignancy. New appearance of focal irregularity of outline in follow-up of a smooth marginated benign lesion is also suspicious of malignant transformation.

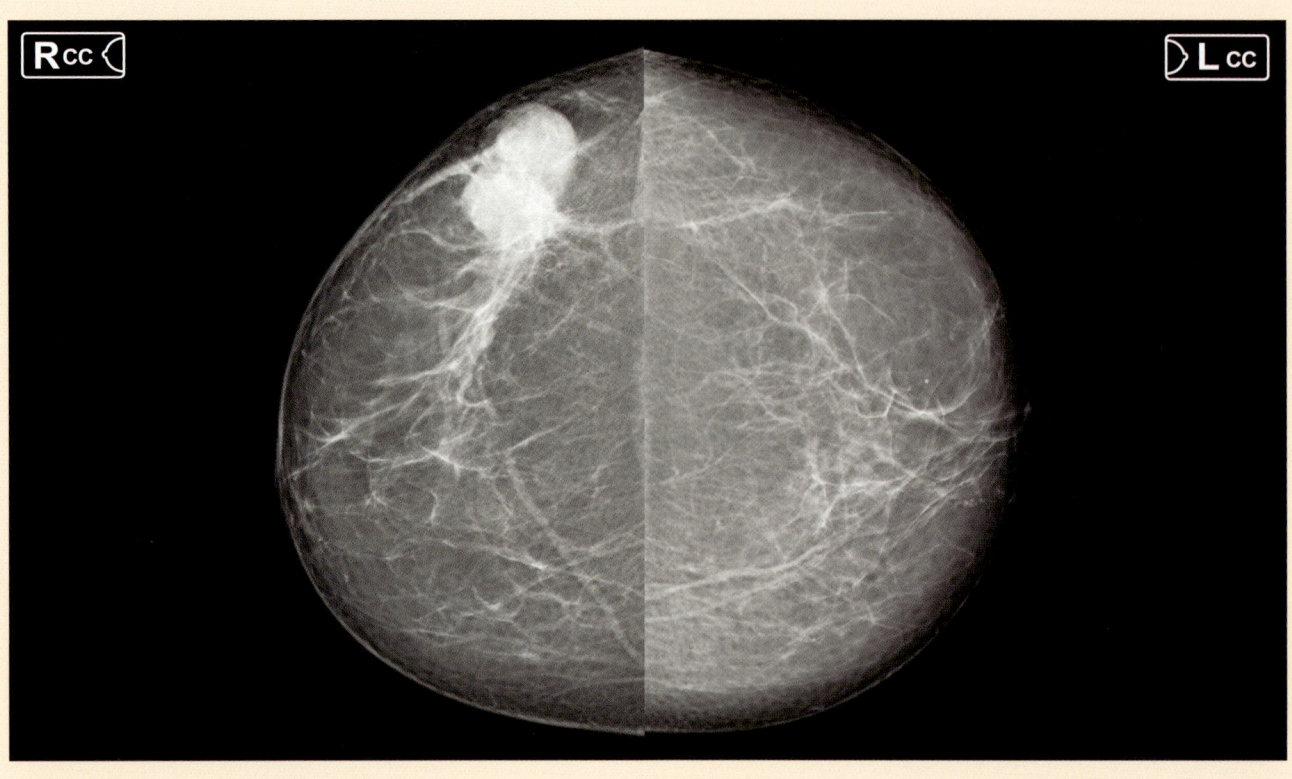

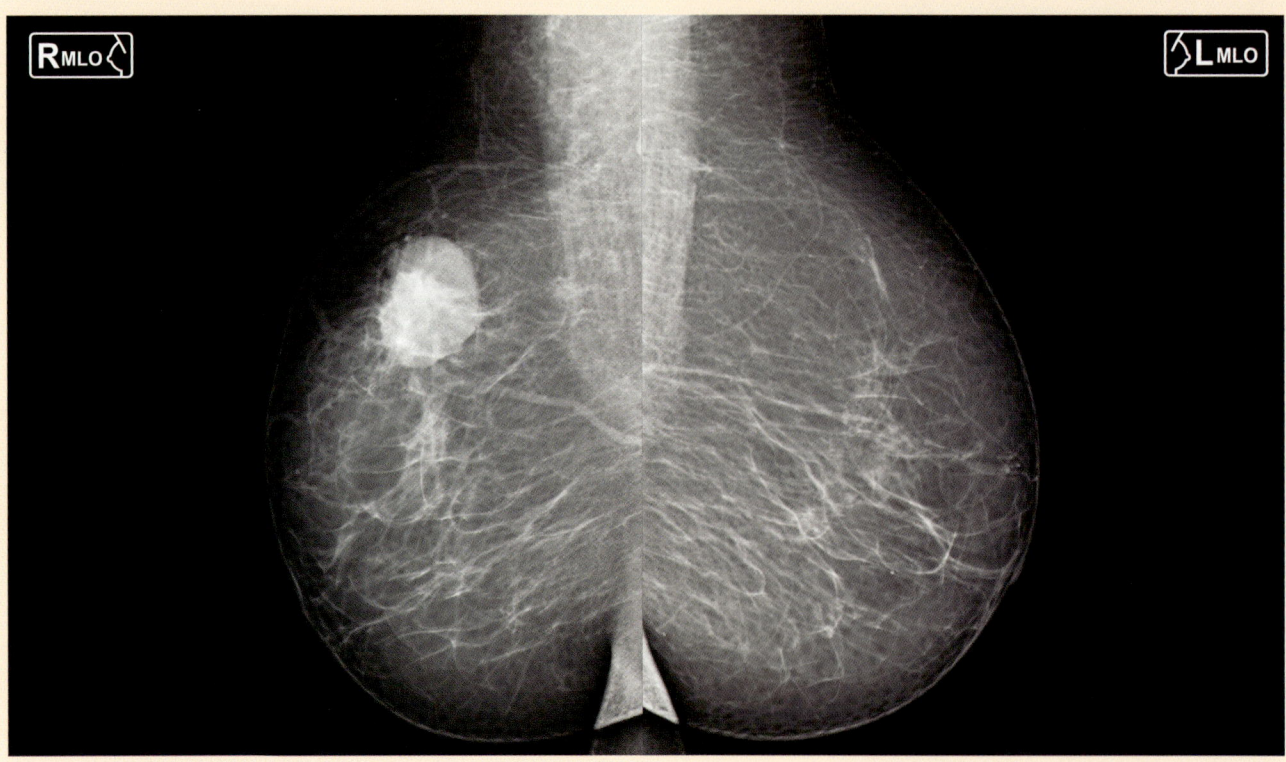

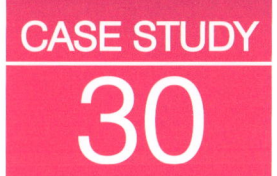

CASE STUDY 30

57-year-old lady presenting with lump in left breast

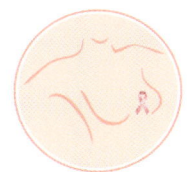

Mammography

ACR Type B density.

Dense rounded lesion of 2.5 cm in size in upper-inner quadrant of left breast showing microlobulation with irregularity of outline. BIRADS V.

USG-guided biopsy positive for malignancy.

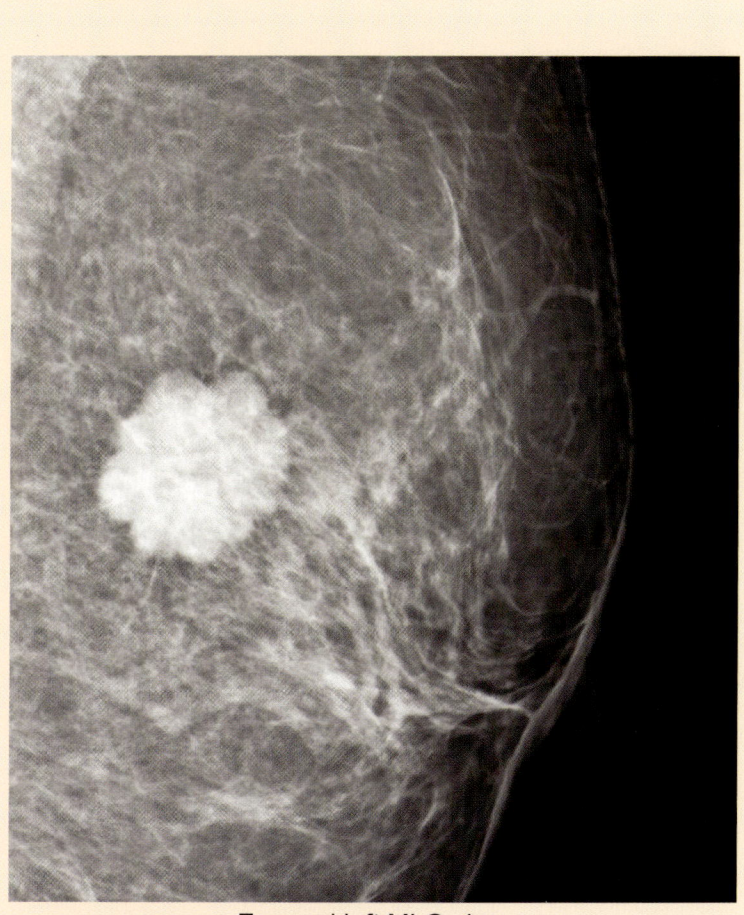

Zoomed left MLO view

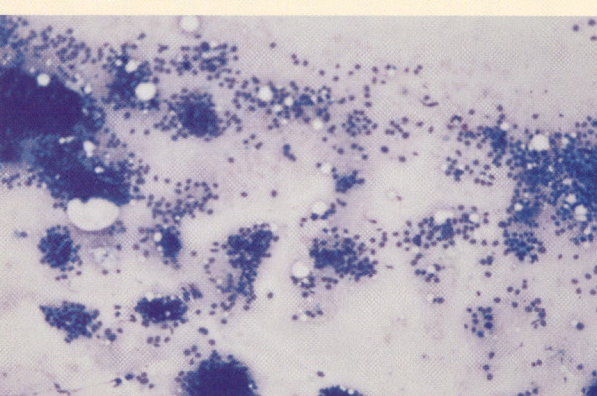

FNAC image

Key Points

Rounded lesions with microlobulations, irregular outline are highly suspicious of underlying malignancy.

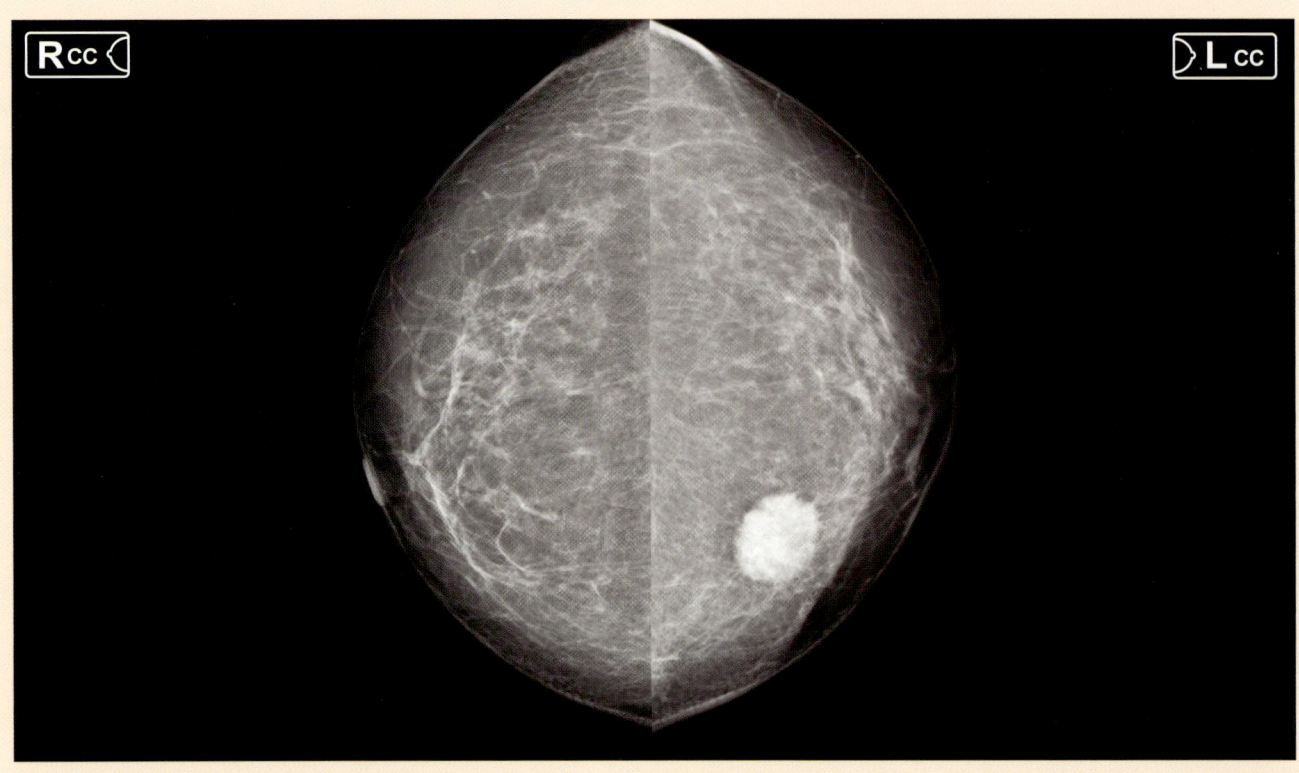

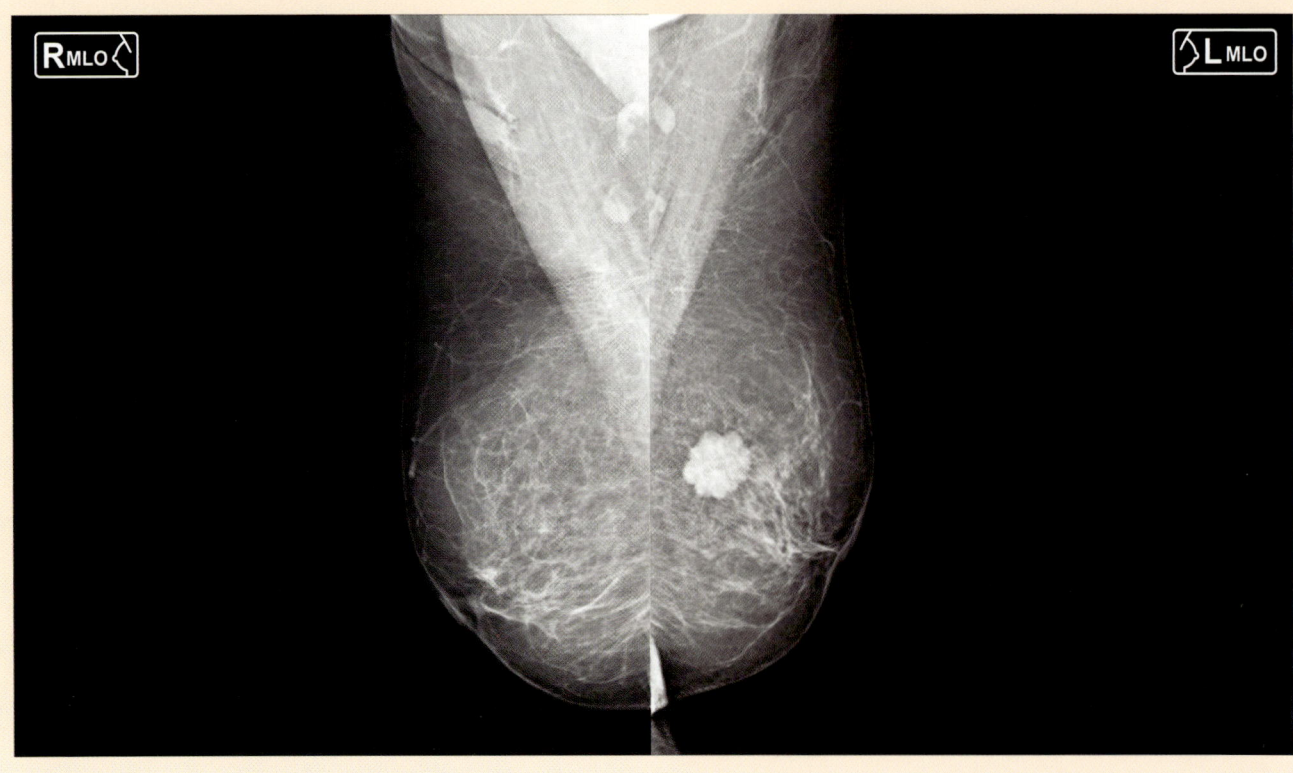

71-year-old lady known case of NHL for routine breast screening

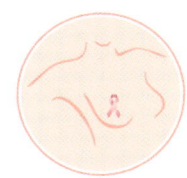

Mammography

ACR Type B density.

A rounded soft tissue lesion of size 1.3 cm in upper-inner quadrant of left breast, showing spiculated outline with associated mild surrounding architectural distortion. BIRADS V.

HPE : Invasive carcinoma of no special type.

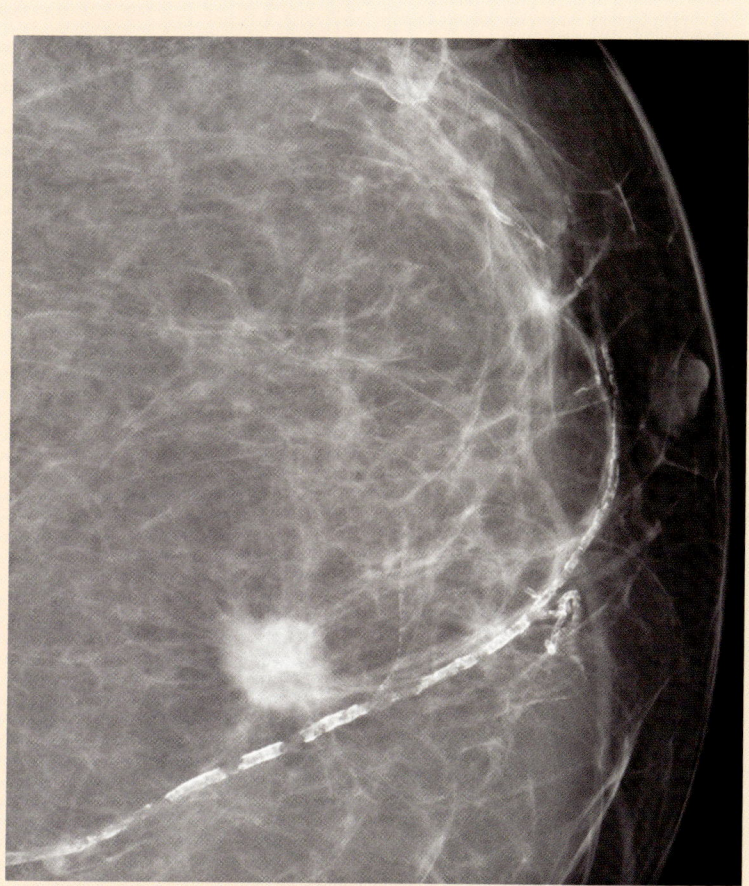

Zoomed left CC view

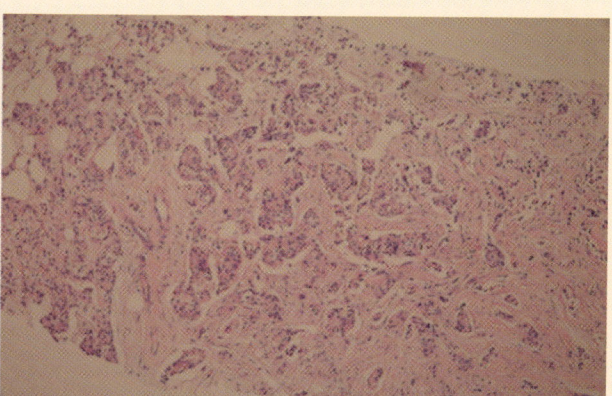

HPE image

Key Points

Rounded spiculated lesions are typical of malignant etiology.

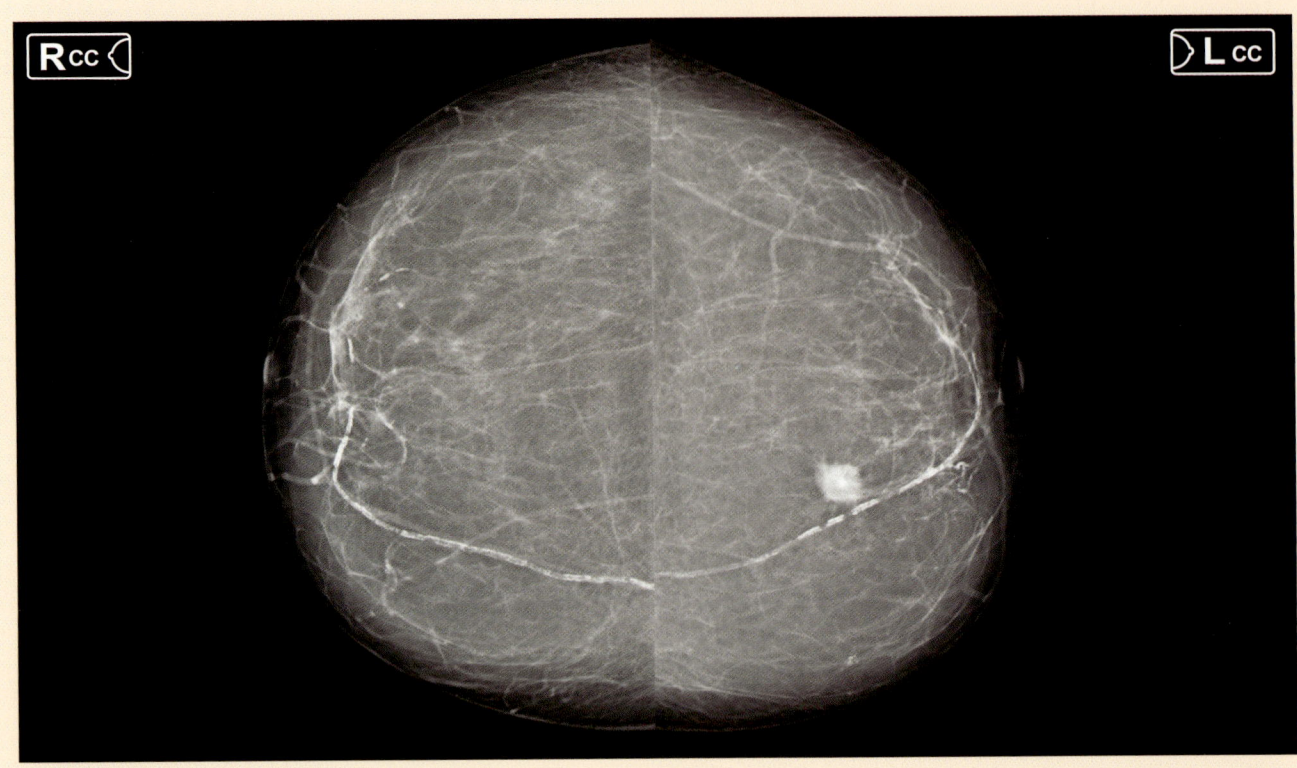

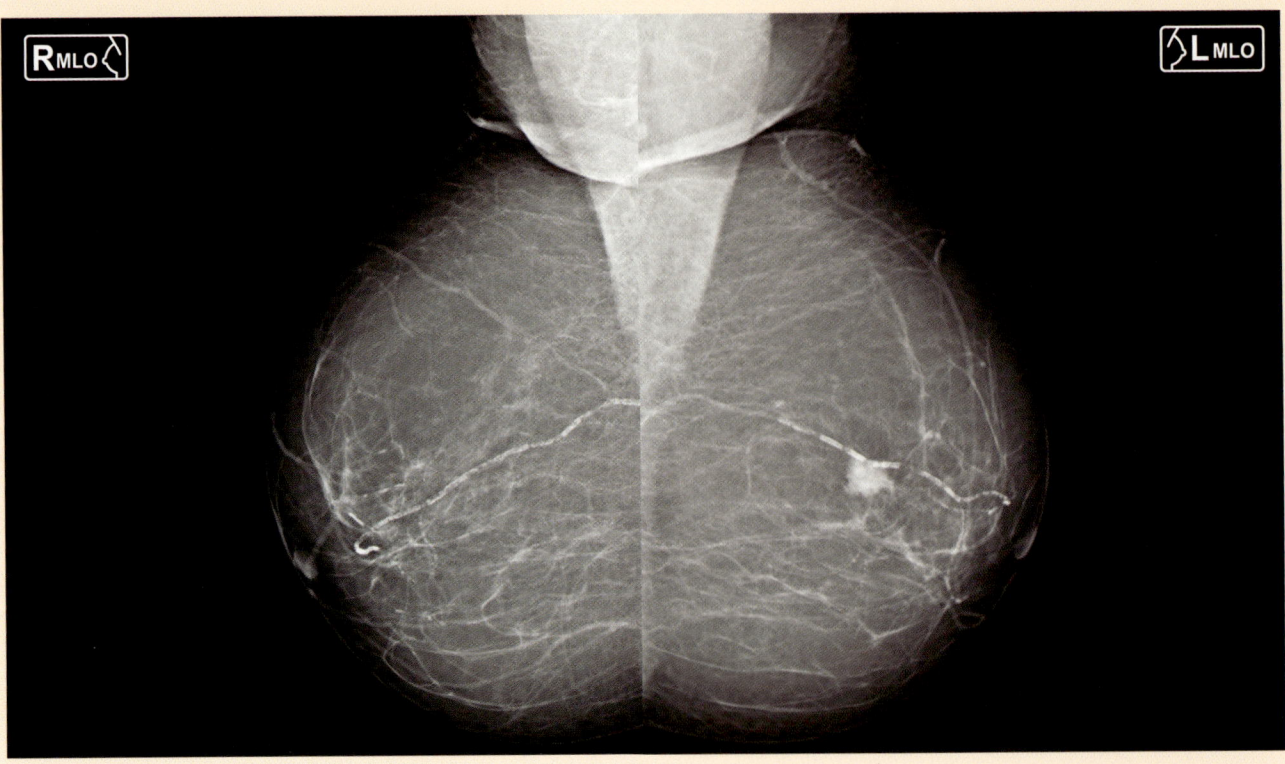

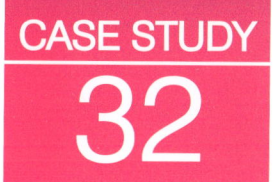
41-year-old lady presenting with lump in right breast

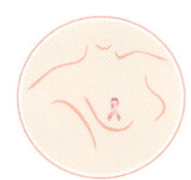

Mammography

ACR Type B density.

Asymmetrical density with architectural distortion in right breast mainly in upper quadrant with diffuse skin thickening. No history of any previous intervention. BIRADS IVc/V.

Suggested USG-guided FNAC/biopsy.

USG-guided FNAC positive for malignant cells.

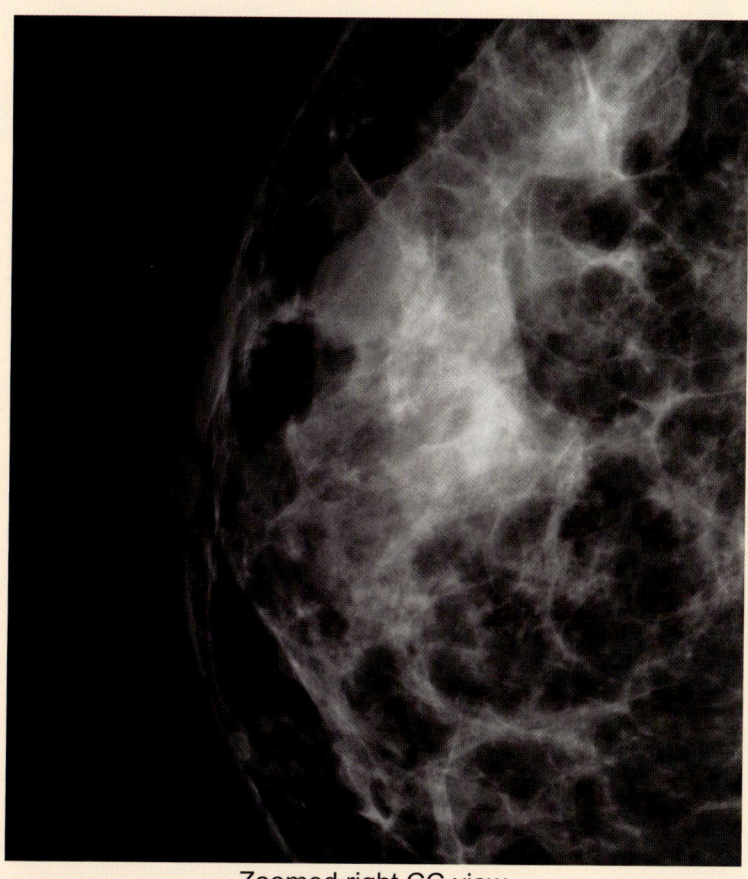

Zoomed right CC view

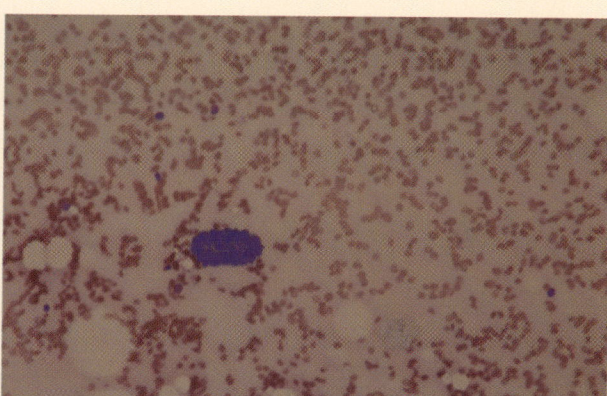

FNAC image

Key Points

Inflammatory carcinoma very often shows diffuse heterogeneous asymmetric density with architectural distortion along with diffuse thickening of overlying skin. HPE correlation should be done.

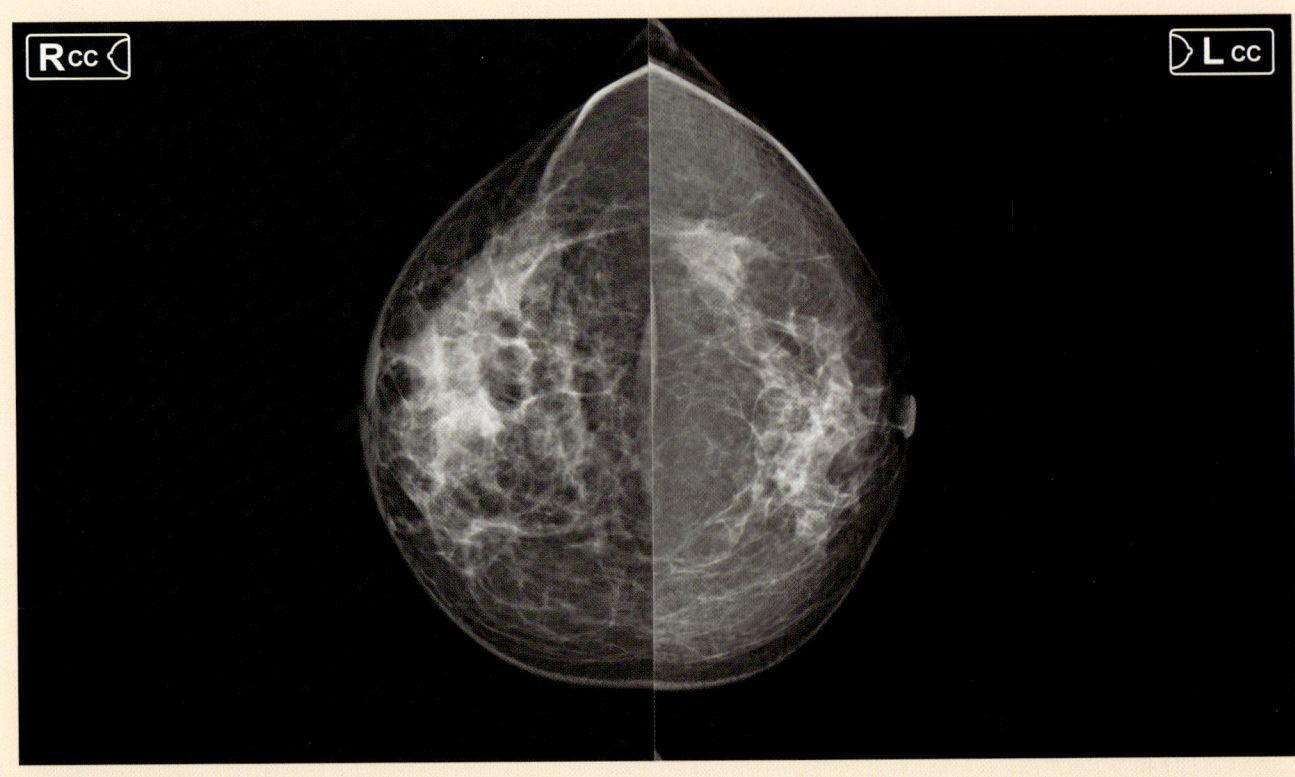

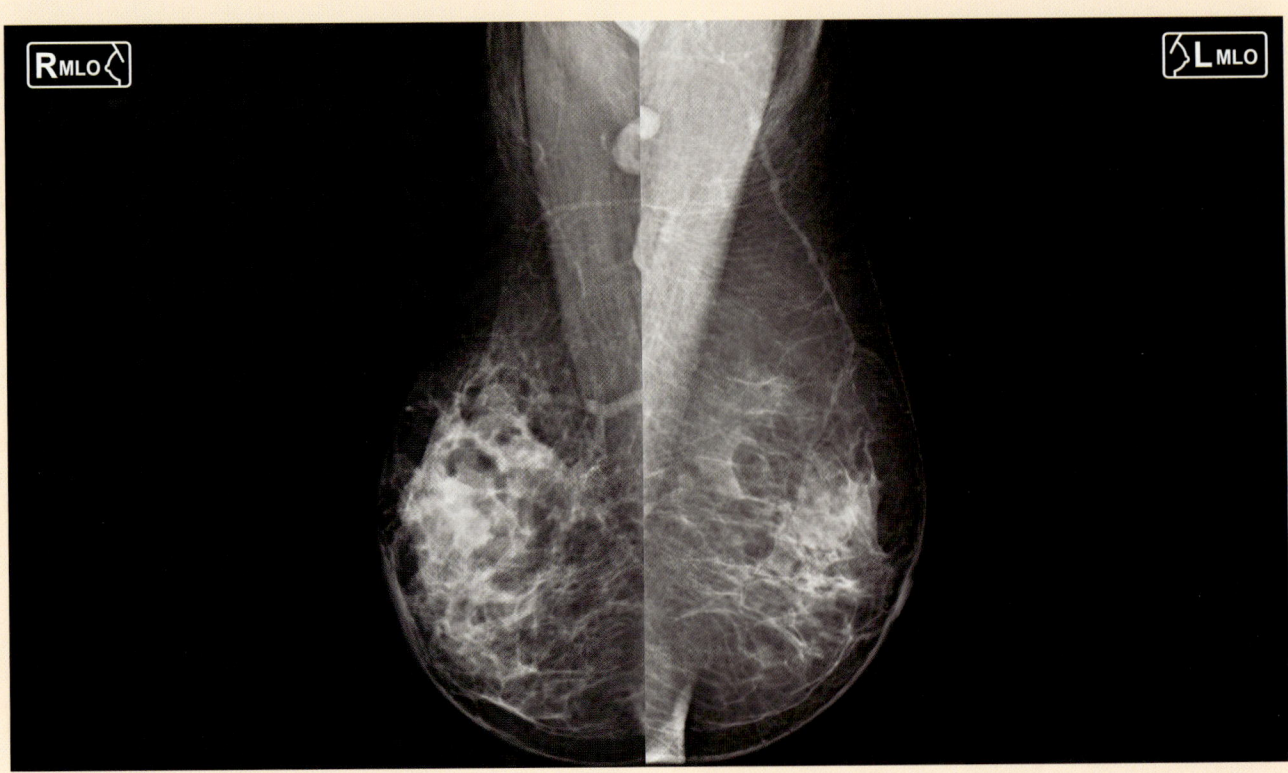

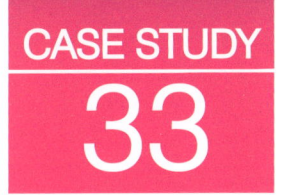
63-year-old lady presenting with right breast lump

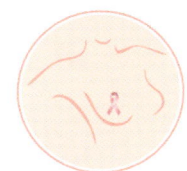

Mammography

Bilateral breasts shows ACR Type C density.

Dense lobulated soft tissue lesion with mild irregularity of outline seen in the upper outer quadrant in right breast.

BIRADS IVc/ V

MRM HPE : Invasive mammary carcinoma

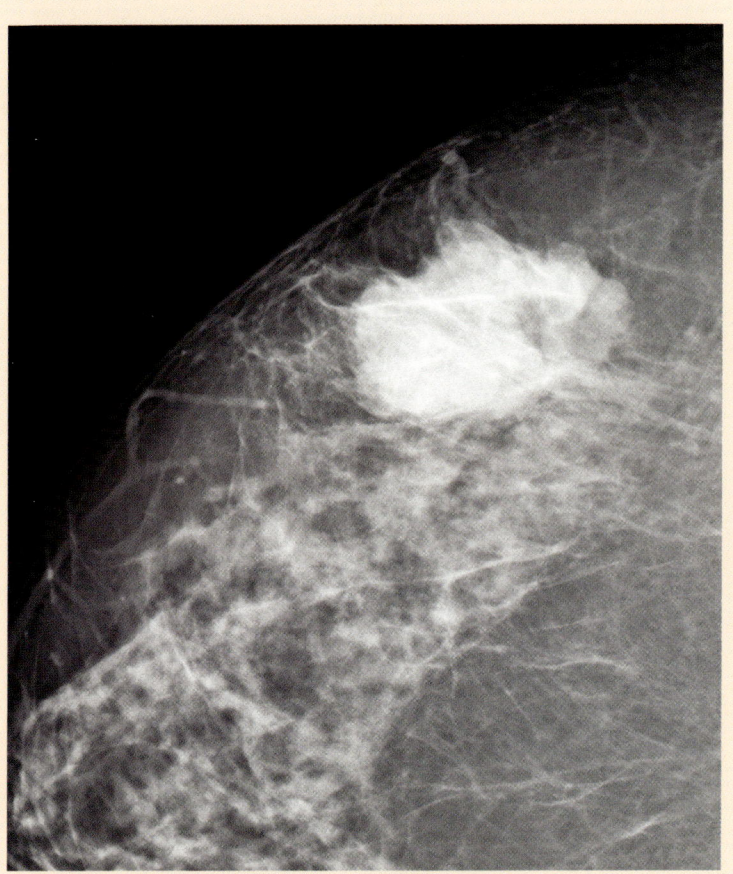

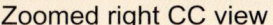
Zoomed right CC view

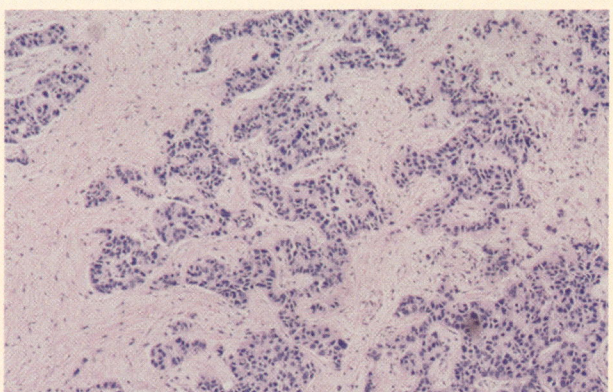
HPE image

Key Points

Malignant masses are often oval in shape, however, unlike benign lesions, the long axis of malignant lesions is in anteroposterior axis, i.e. malignant lesions are taller than wider. The other sinister feature in this case is the high density of the lesion.

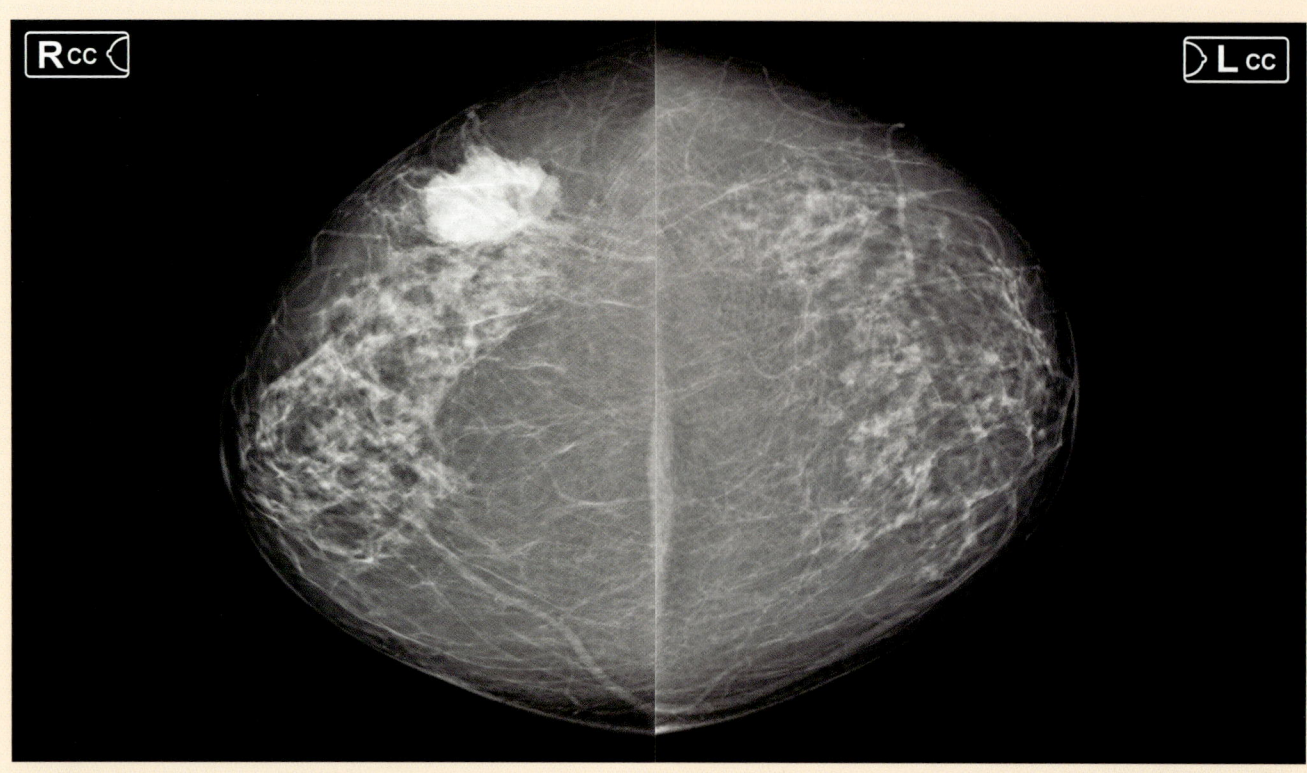

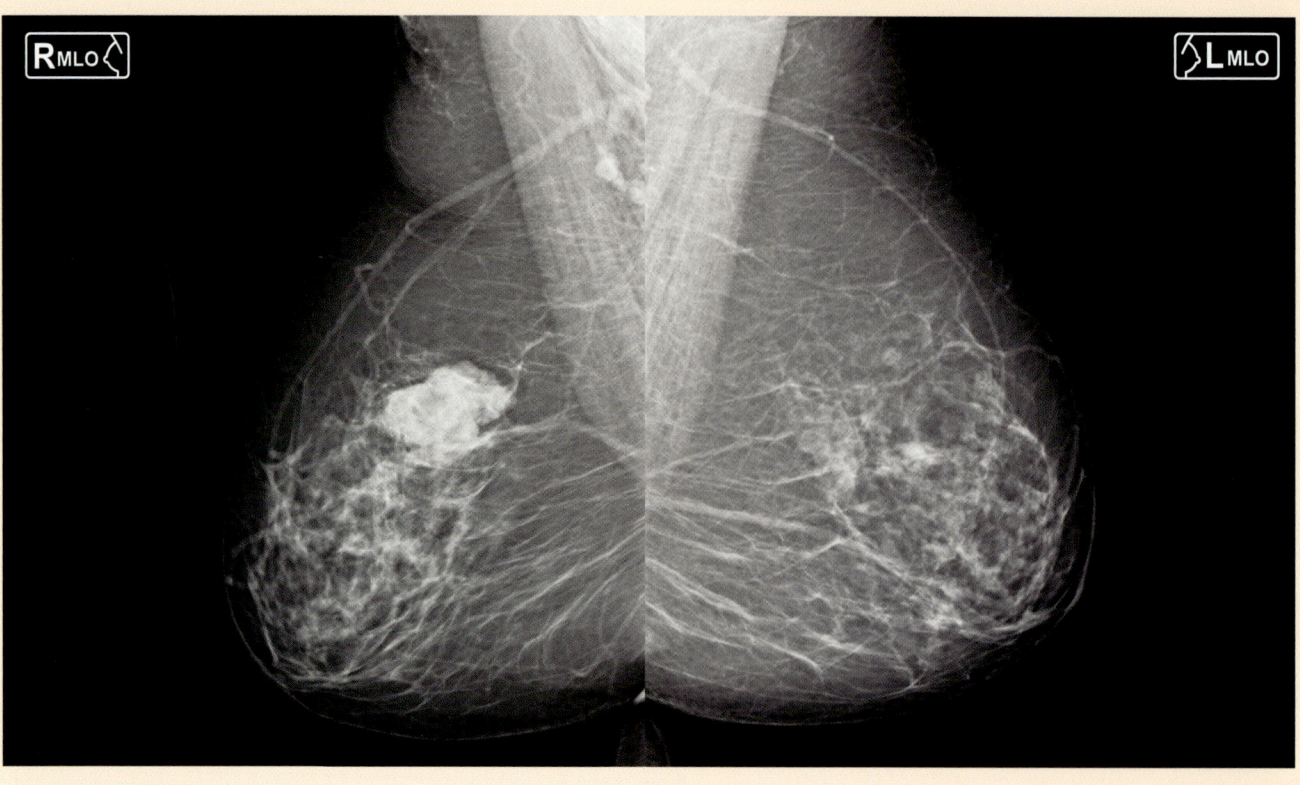

66-year-old lady presenting with lump in right breast

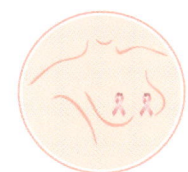

Mammography

ACR Type A density.

Spiculated soft tissue mass lesion of size 2.3 cm in upper quadrant of right breast with another spiculated soft tissue mass lesion of 1.3 cm in the central quadrant of left breast. B/L breast BIRADS V lesions. Suggested HPE correlation.

HPE: Invasive mammary carcinoma of no special type in both breast lesions.

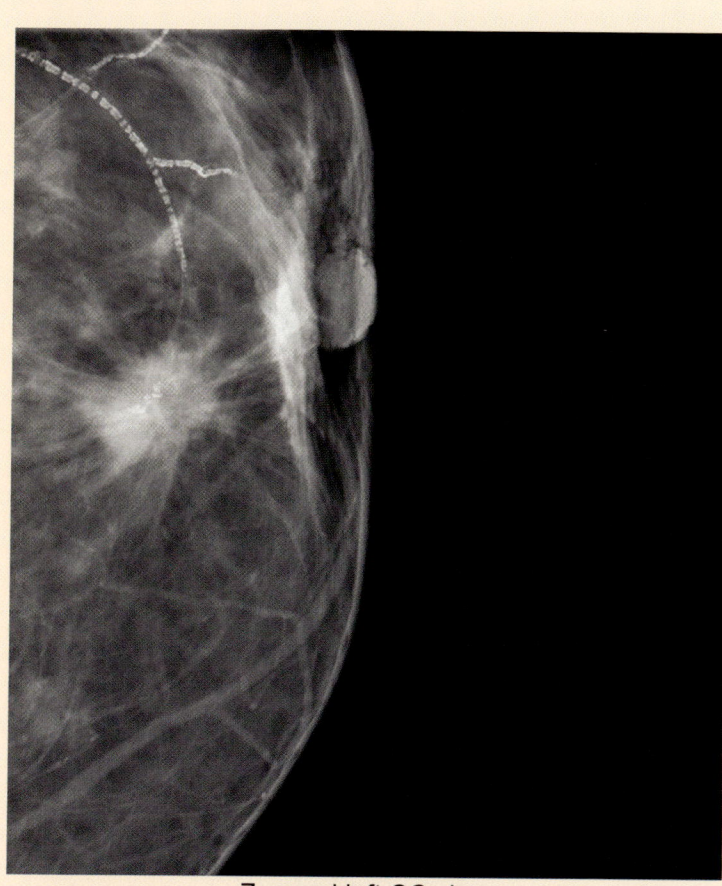

Zoomed left CC view

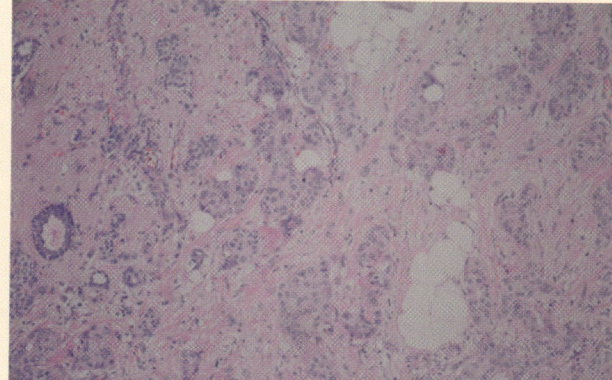

HPE left breast lesion

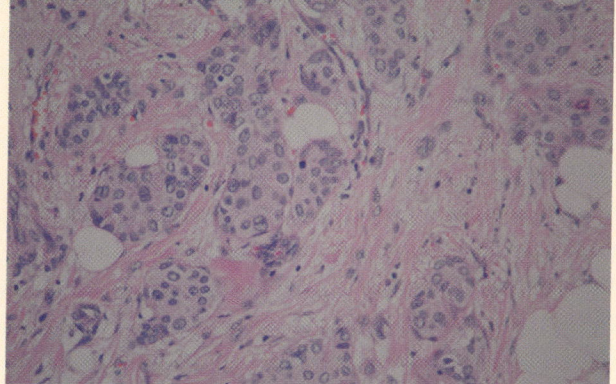

HPE right breast lesion

Key Points

Mammography should always be done for both breasts even in the clinical setting of malignant appearing mass lesion in one breast with no clinical abnormality in the other.

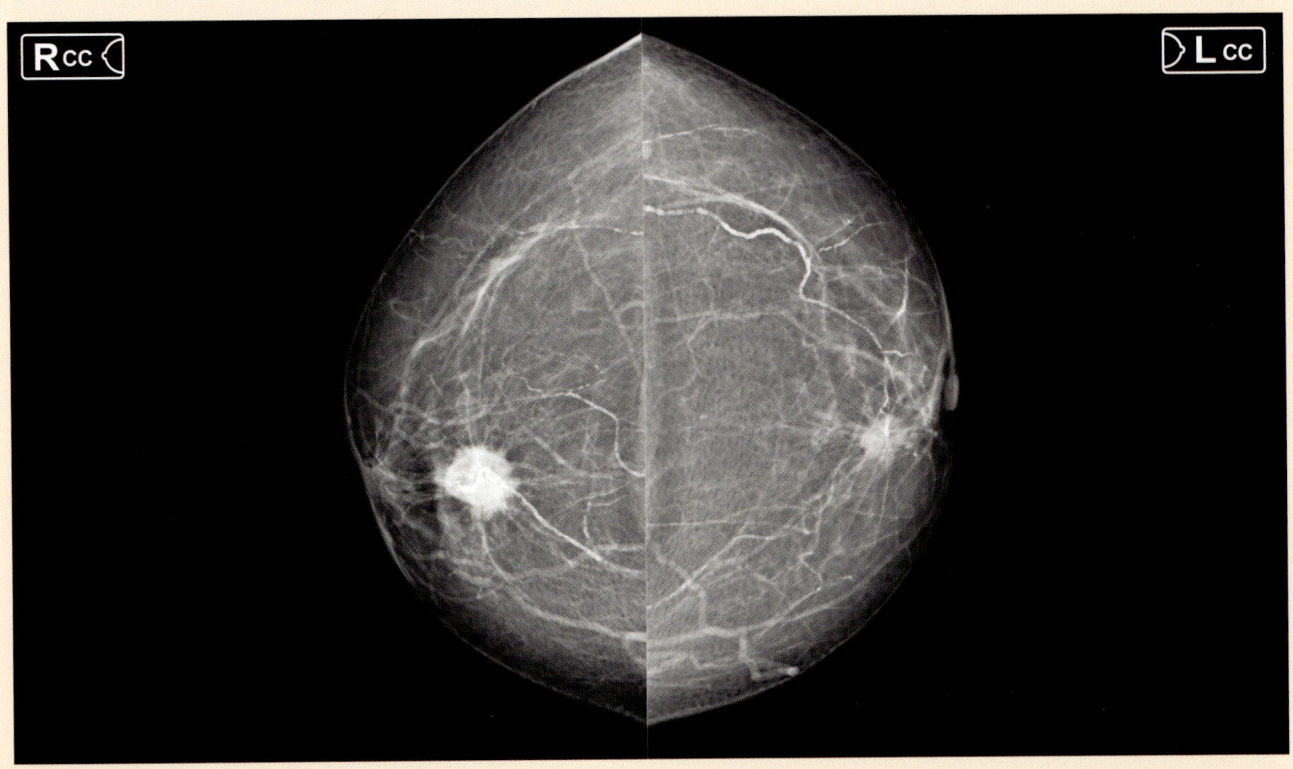

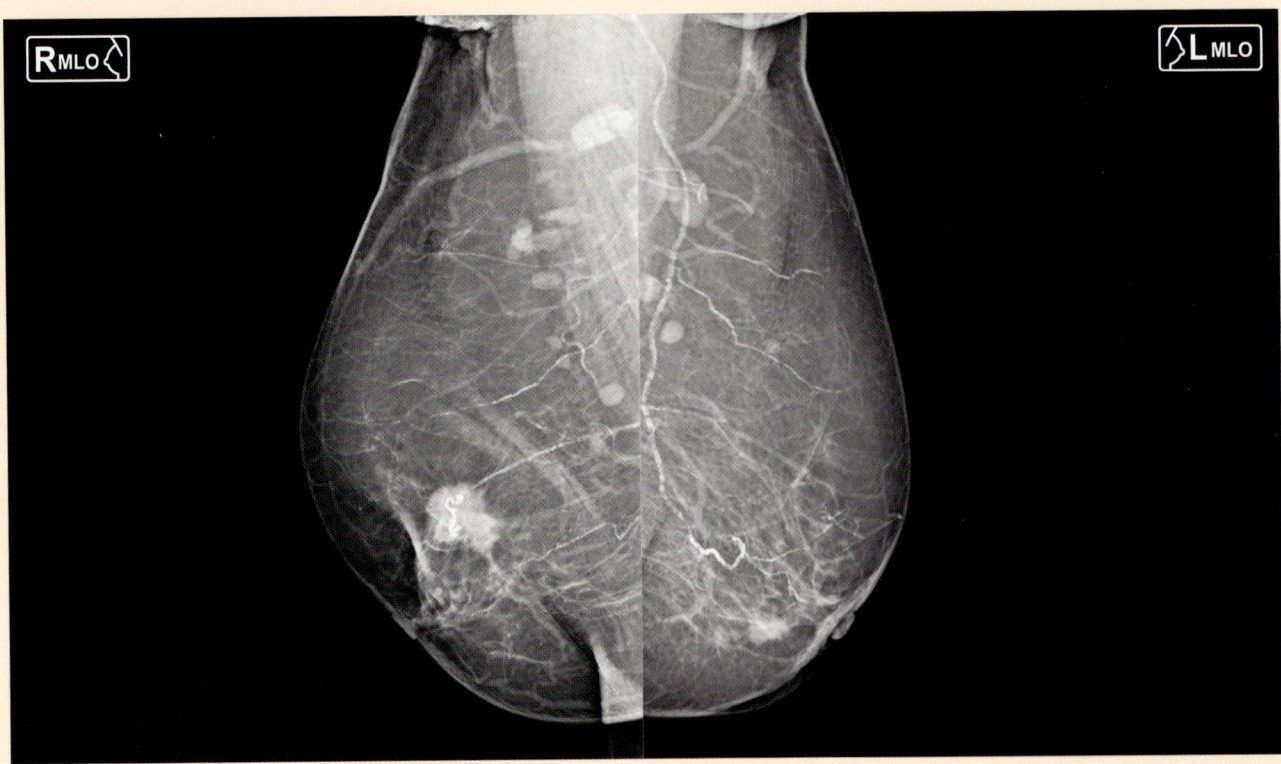

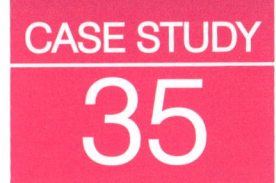

64-year-old lady, 2 yrs post left MRM for Ca left breast, for screening

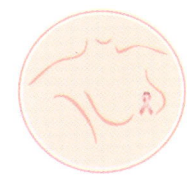

Mammography

Small cluster of pleomorphic microcalcifications in upper quadrant of right breast. The abnormality was not seen in previous outside mammography done 1yr earlier. BIRADS IVc. Suggested stereotactic biopsy.

Stereotactic biposy of right breast lesion was positive for malignancy.

MRM HPE: DCIS with no invasive component

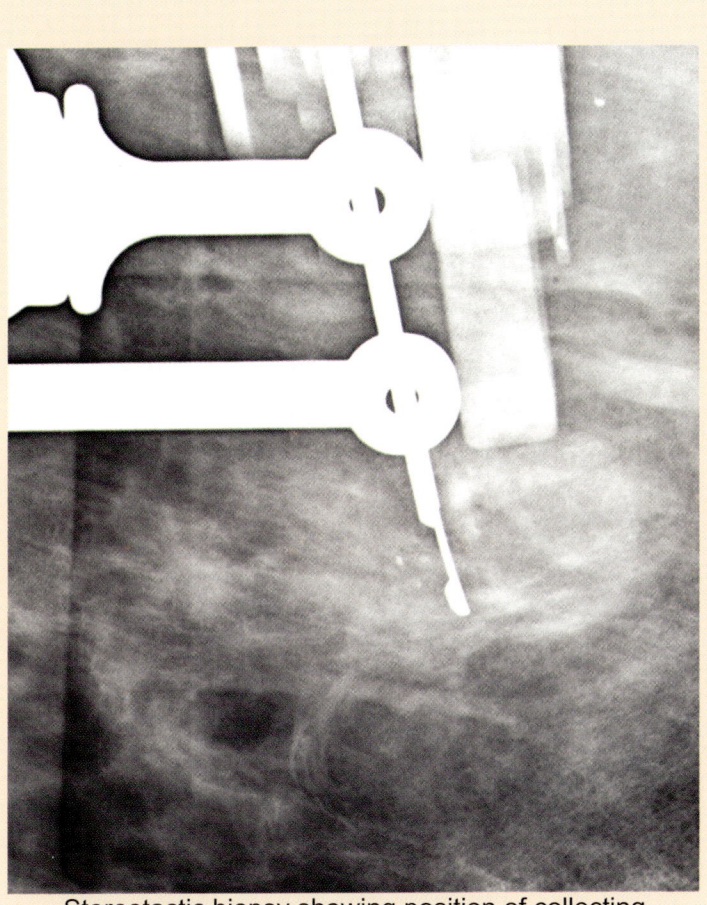

Stereotactic biopsy showing position of collecting chamber in relation to the lesion

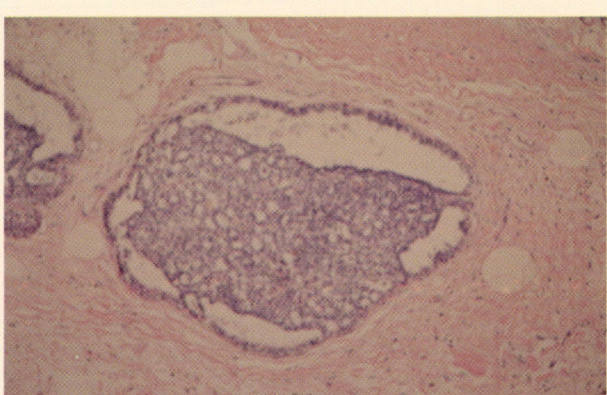

HPE image

Key Points

Clustered pleomorphic microcalcifications are suspicious for underlying malignancy. These are many times not seen on USG, often with no corresponding suspicious abnormality on MRI and these imaging can be falsely re-assuring. Stereotactic biopsy of the clustered microcalcification should be the next step.

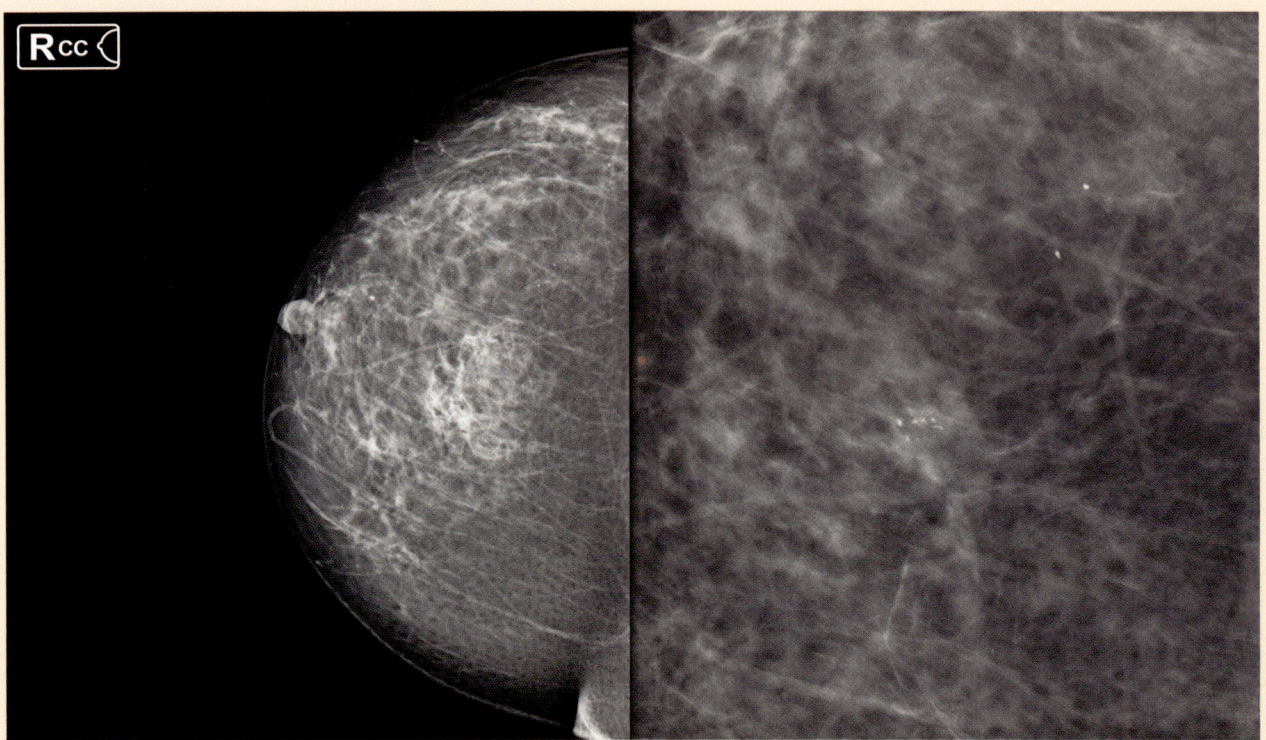

Spot magnification view of right breast lesion

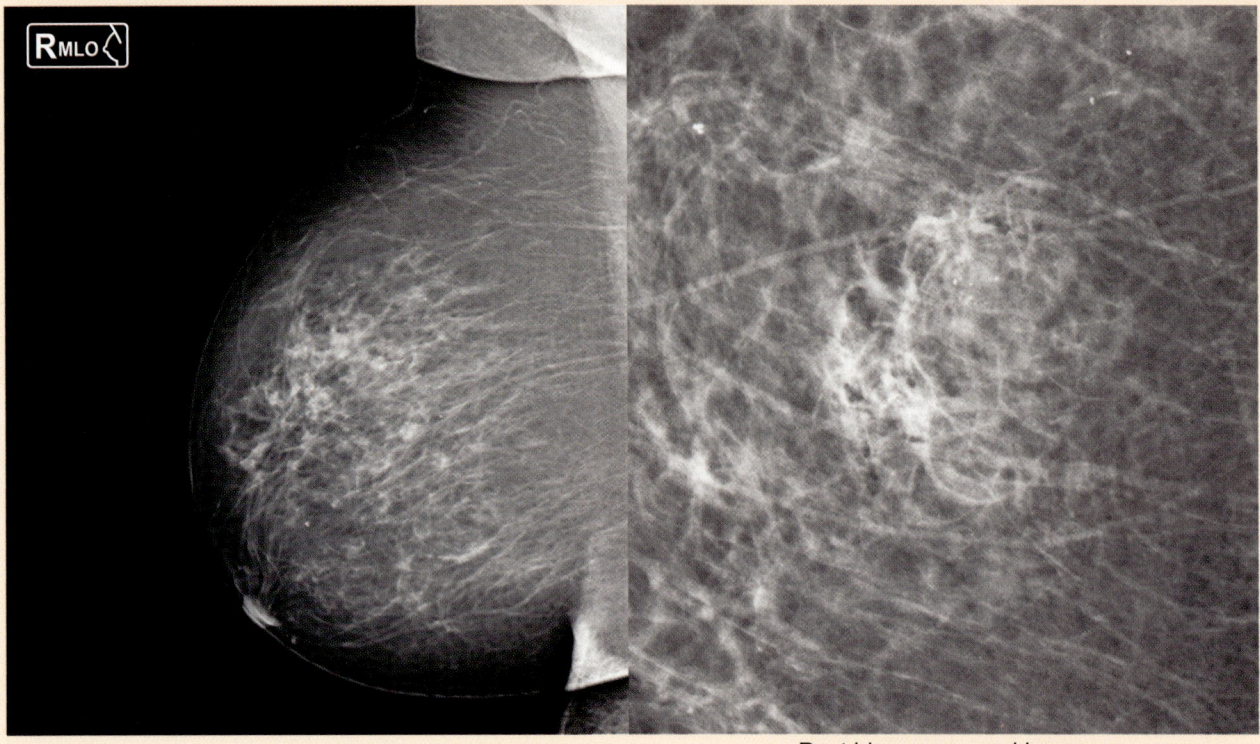

Post biopsy zoomed image

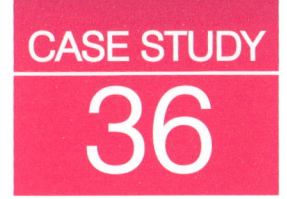
53-year-old lady with retracted left nipple

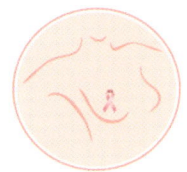

Mammography

ACR Type C density.

Spiculated lesion with internal polymorphic micro-calcifications in central quardant with architectural distortions.

Retracted nipple and diffuse skin thickening.

BIRADS V, suggested HPE correlation.

USG-guided biopsy: Invasive mammary carcinoma.

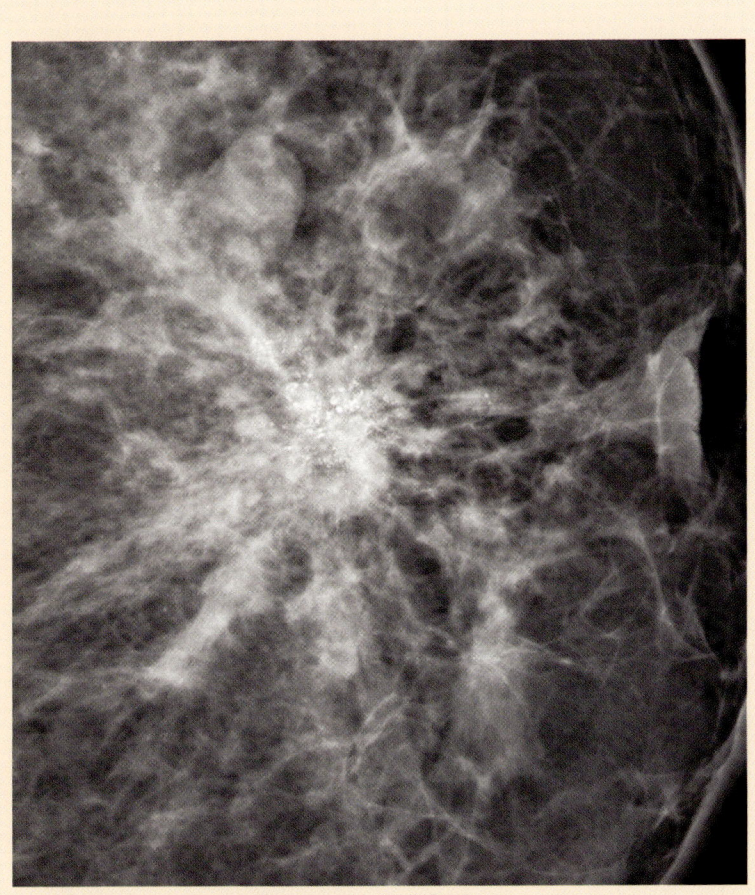

Zoomed left CC view

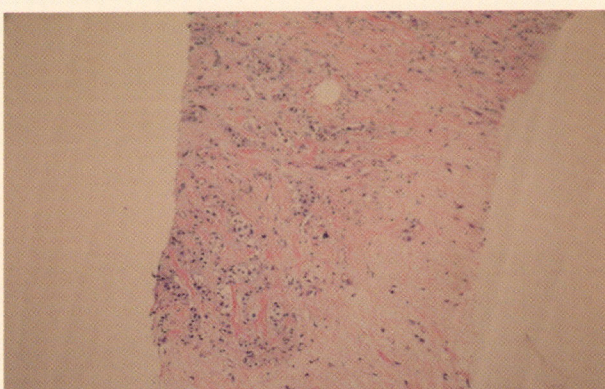

HPE image

Key Points

Nipple retraction of recent onset should be viewed with high clinical suspicion even in the absence of any palpable clinical lump. Mammography evaluation should be done at the earliest.

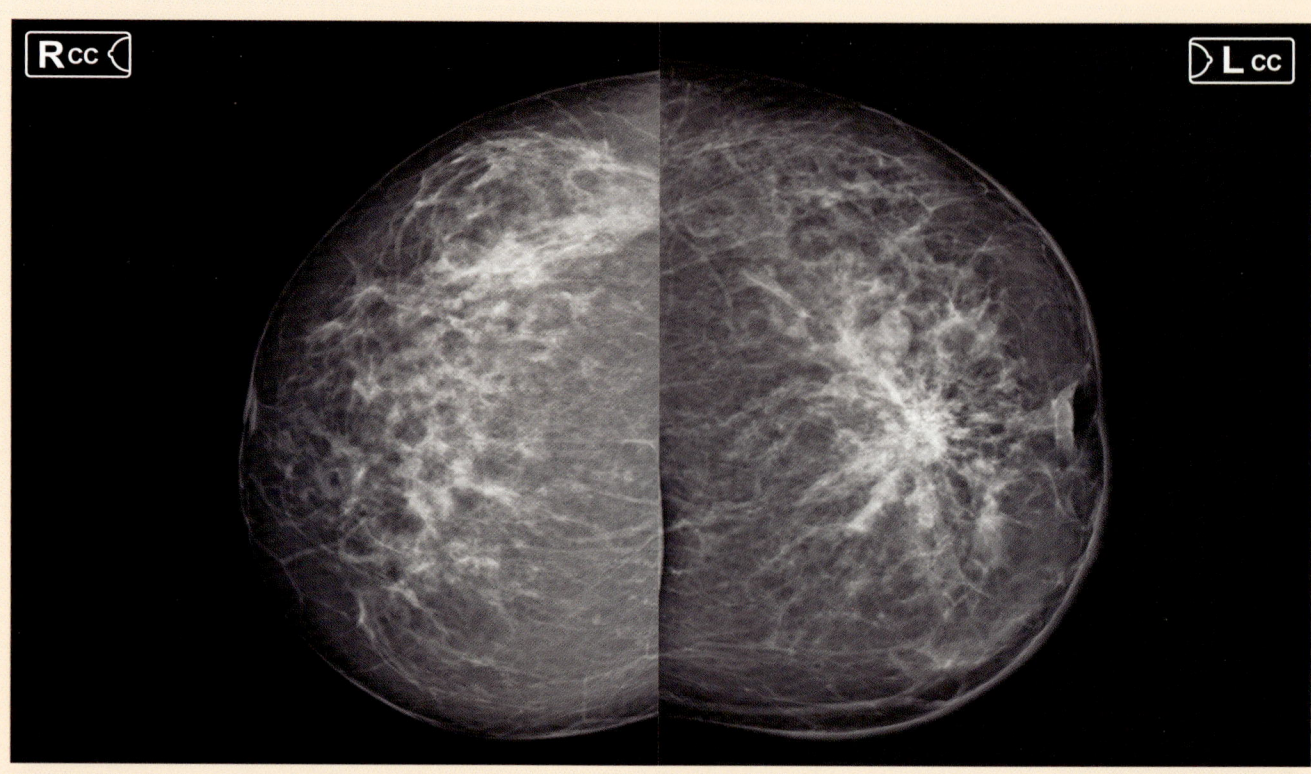

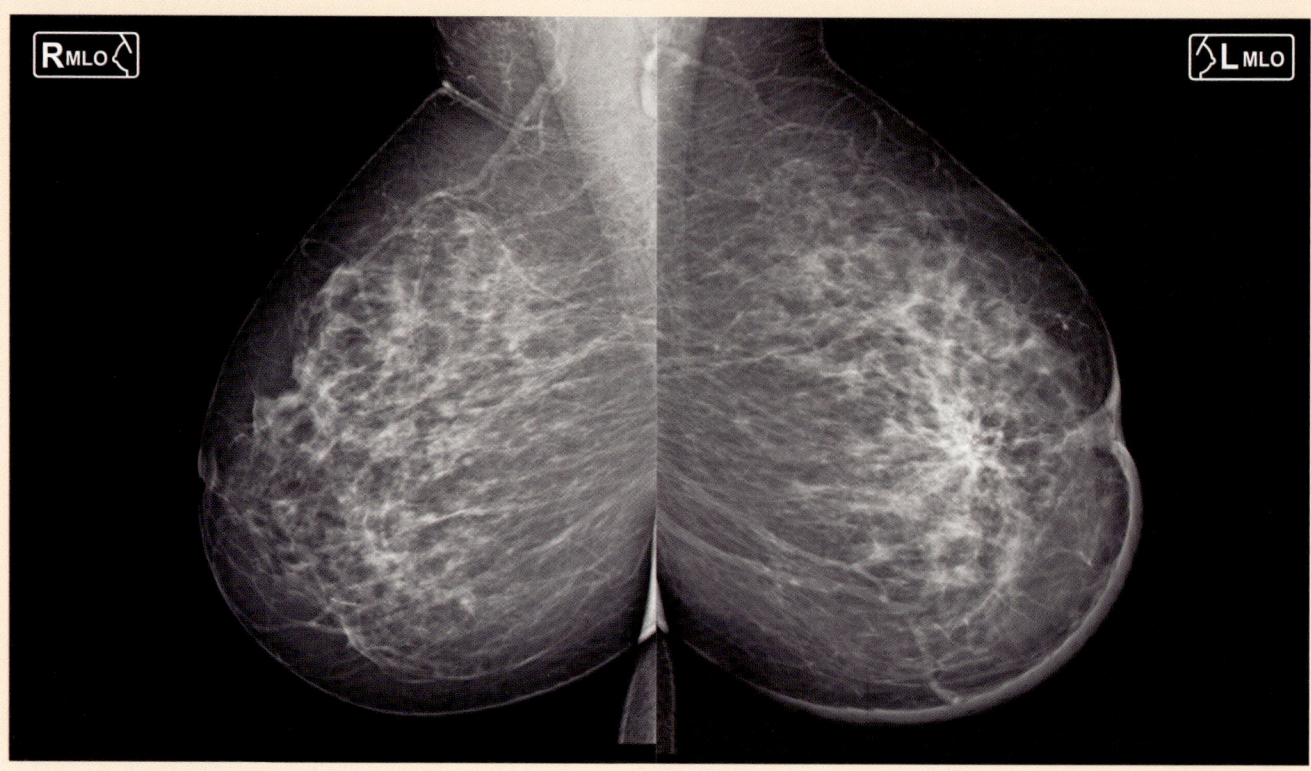

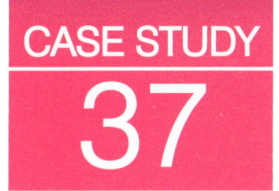

50-year-old lady with right breast lump

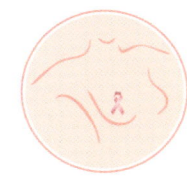

Mammography

ACR Type B density.

Multiple branching tubular/nodular soft tissue densities in the central quadrant with diffuse architectural distortion, thickened stroma in right breast with mildly retracted nipple and diffuse skin thickening. A few microcalcifications seen scattered in right breast with a few enlarged right axillary nodes. BIRADS V (features suggesting inflammatory carcinoma)

USG-guided biopsy from right breast lesion revealed invasive mammary carcinoma of no special type.

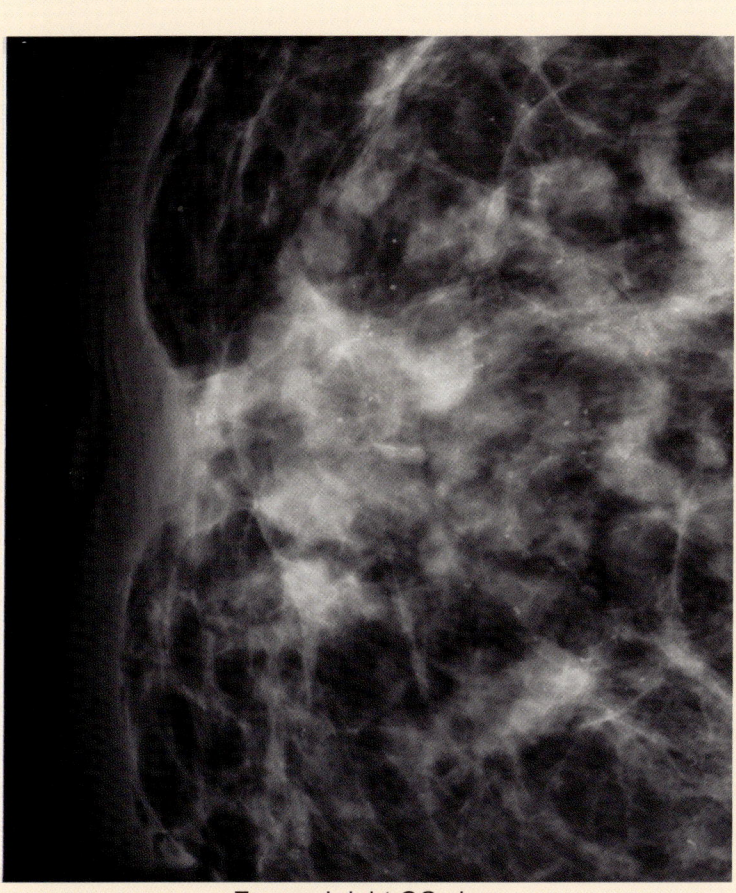

Zoomed right CC view

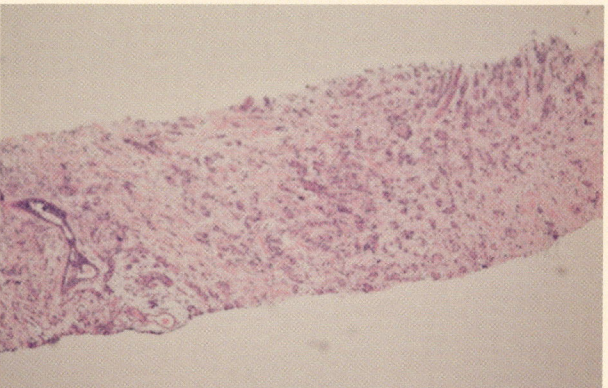

HPE image

Key Points

Diffuse stromal thickening with architectural distortion, ductal soft tissue opacities, retracted nipple and skin thickening are hallmarks of advanced/ inflammatory breast cancer.

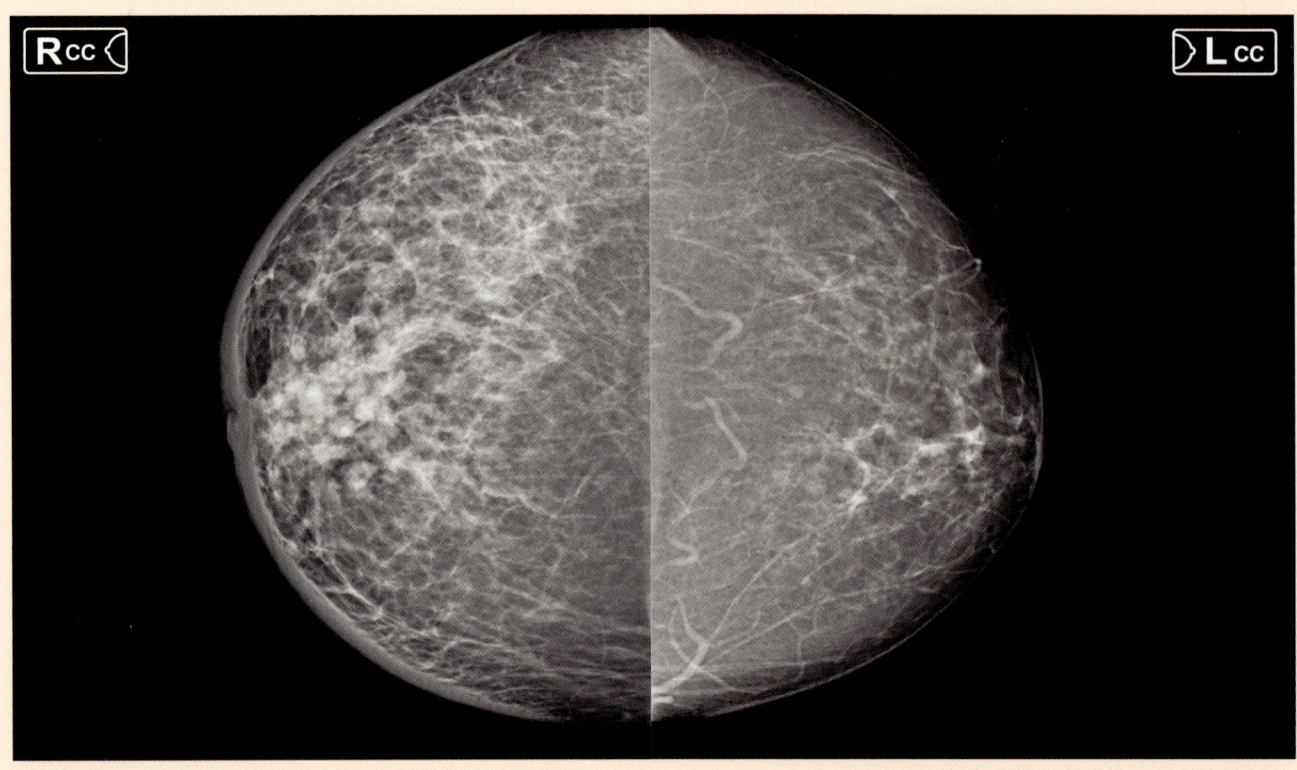

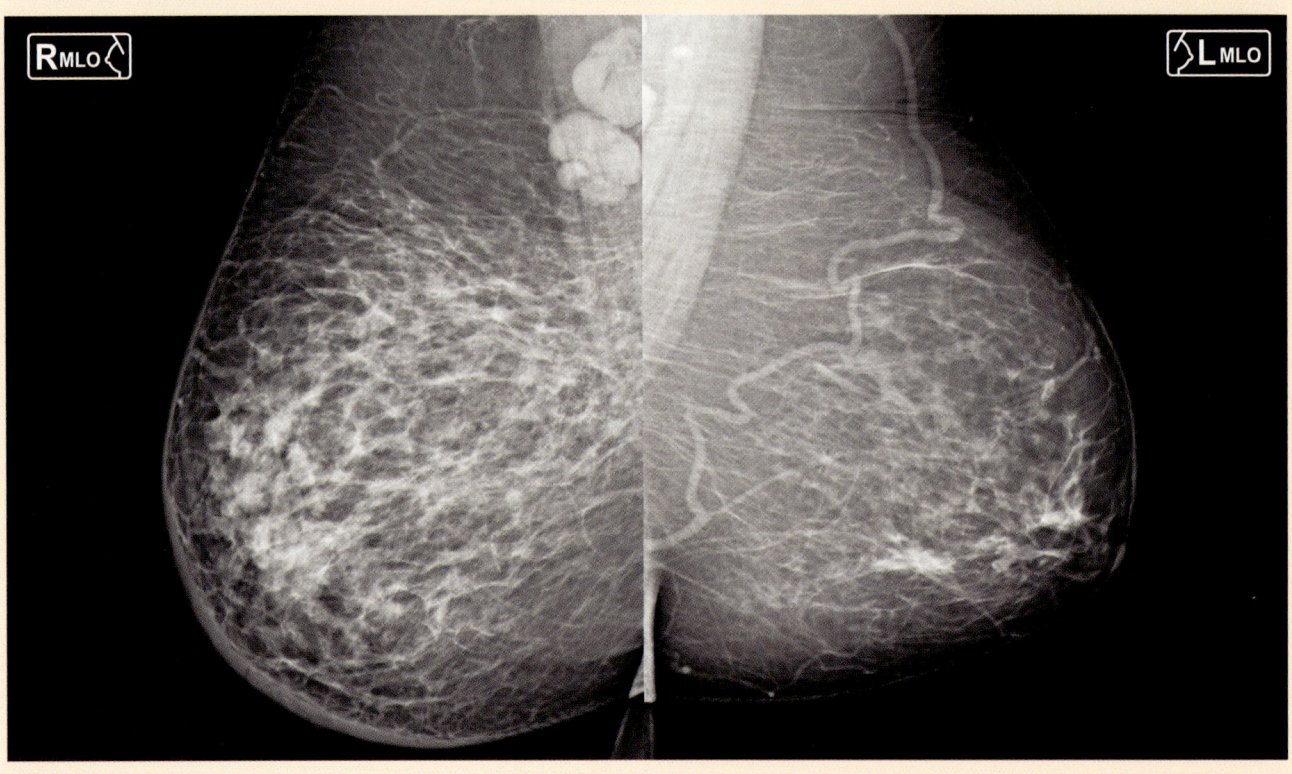

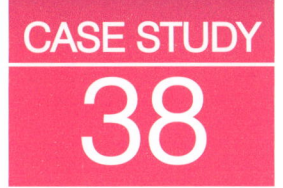
52-year-old lady for screening

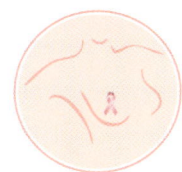

Mammography

ACR Type B density.

Clustered microcalcifications in the outer quadrant of left breast, apparently in segmental/ductal distribution with no abnormality in right breast. Spot magnification view obtained for left breast. Suggested stereotactic biopsy.

Stereotactic biopsy of left breast lesion showed no evidence of DCIS/malignancy. Further discussions in oncoradiology meet suggested to offer lumpectomy on view of high suspicion of malignancy in mammography.

Lumpectomy HPE : DCIS of 4.5 x 3 x 2 cm size.

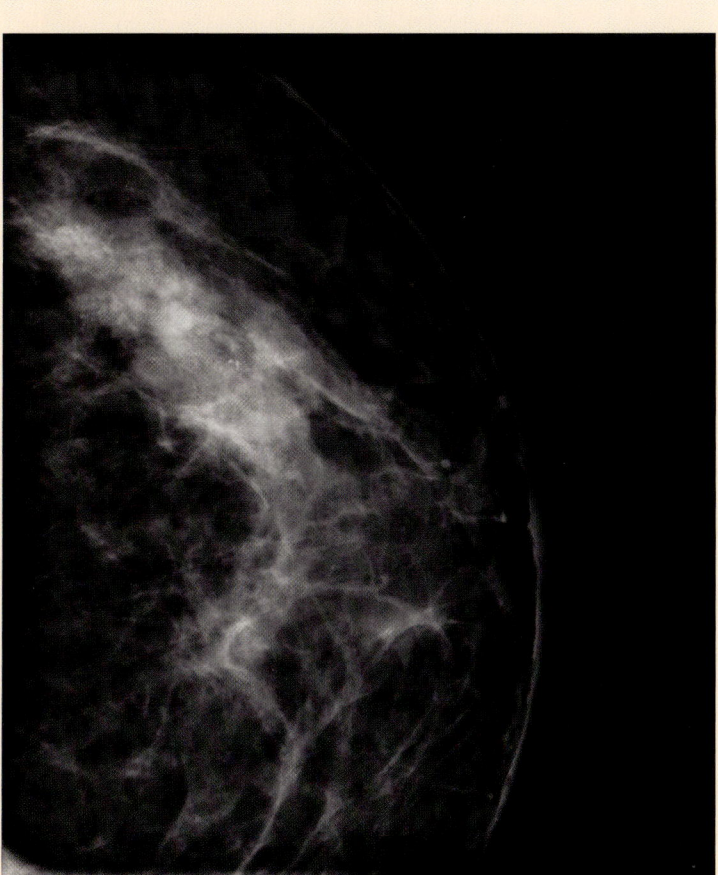

Spot magnification for outer quadrant left breast

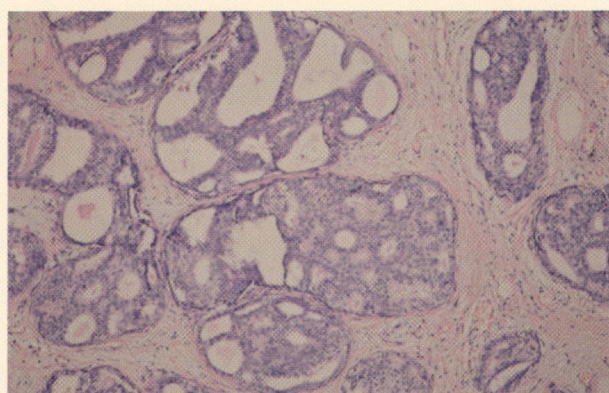

HPE image

Key Points

Microcalcifications in ductal/segmental pattern raises high suspicion of malignancy. Trucut core biopsy may occasionally be negative. We should consider offering a repeat biopsy/lumpectomy after wire localization for complete work-up.

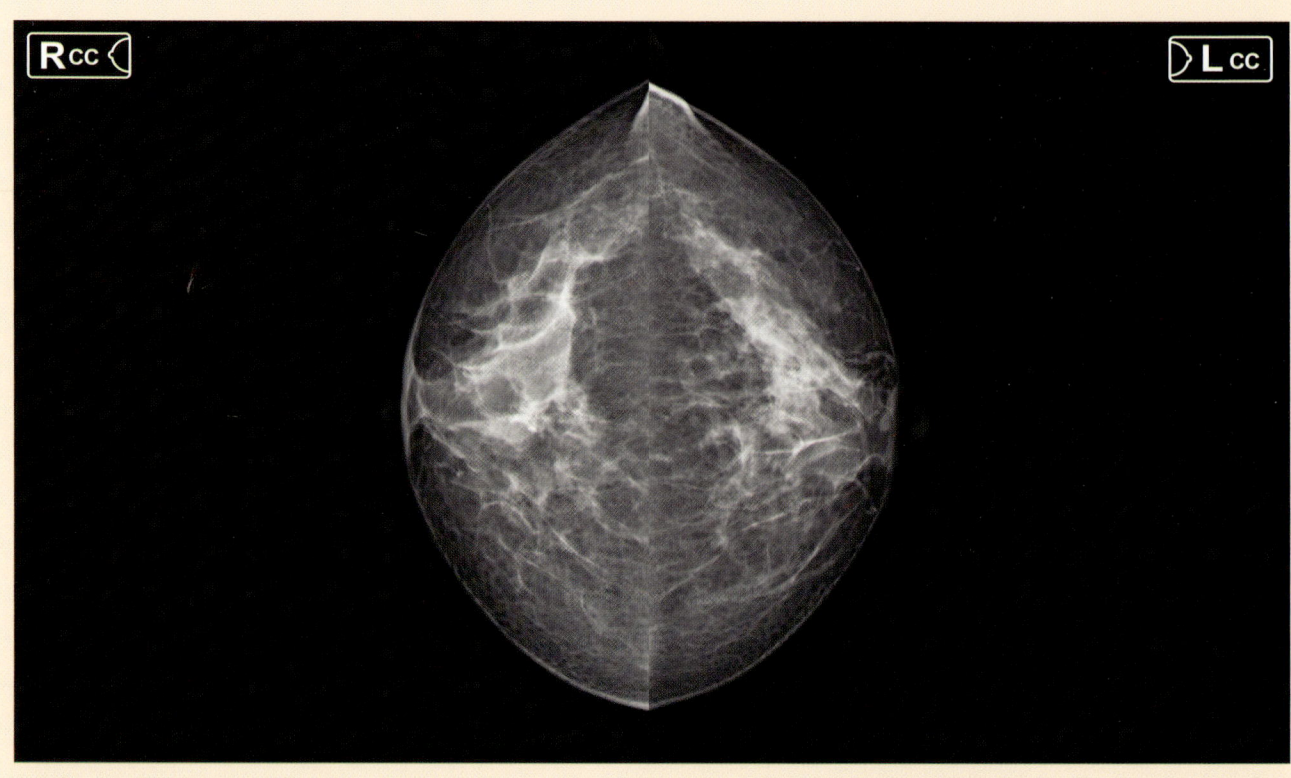

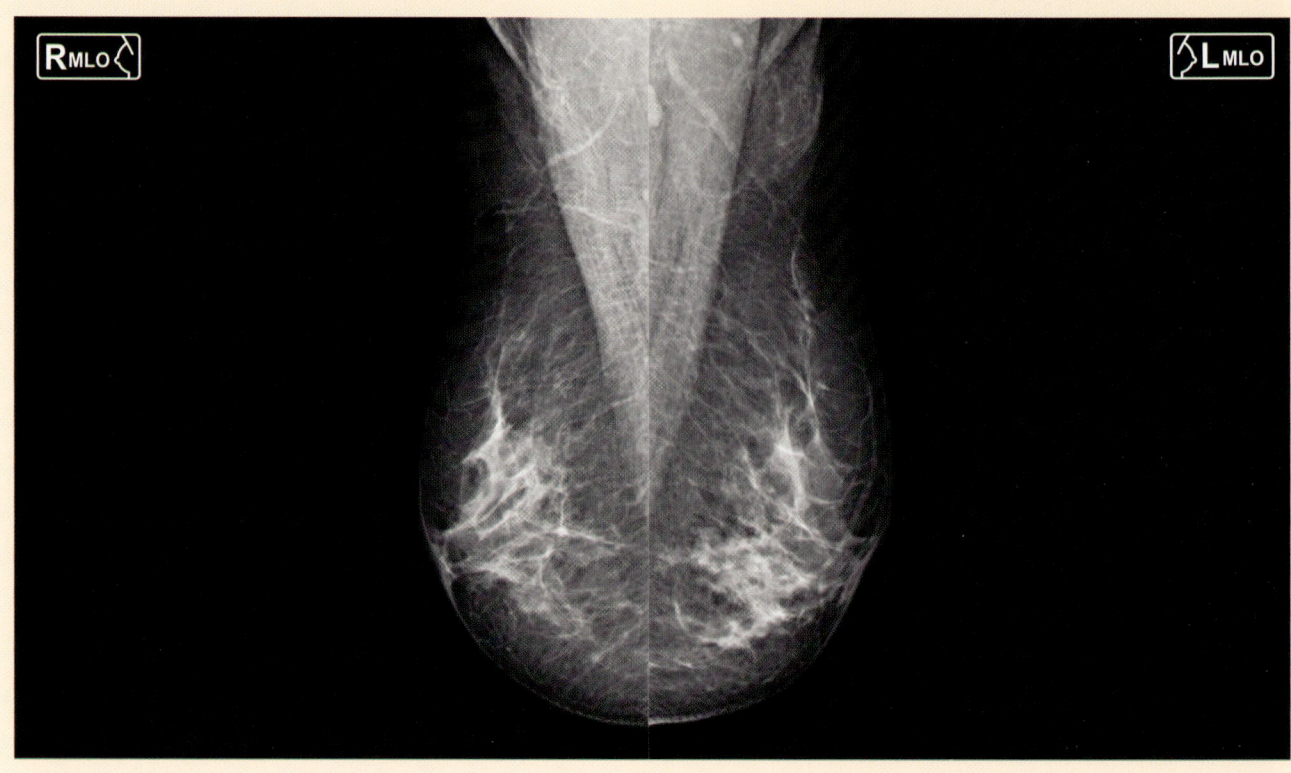

50-year-old lady with lump in right breast

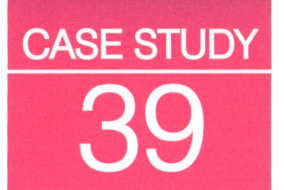
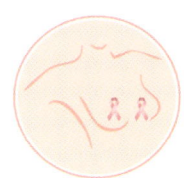

Mammography

ACR Type B density.

Spiculated soft tissue mass lesion with surrounding architectural distortion and internal pleomorphic micro-, macro-calcifications in upper outer quadrant of right breast. Soft tissue opacity with clustered microcalcifications in upper-outer quadrant of left breast. Right breast BIRADS V. Left breast lesion BIRADS IVc.

Left breast lumpectomy HPE: DCIS.

Right breast lumpectomy HPE: Invasive mammary carcinoma of no special type.

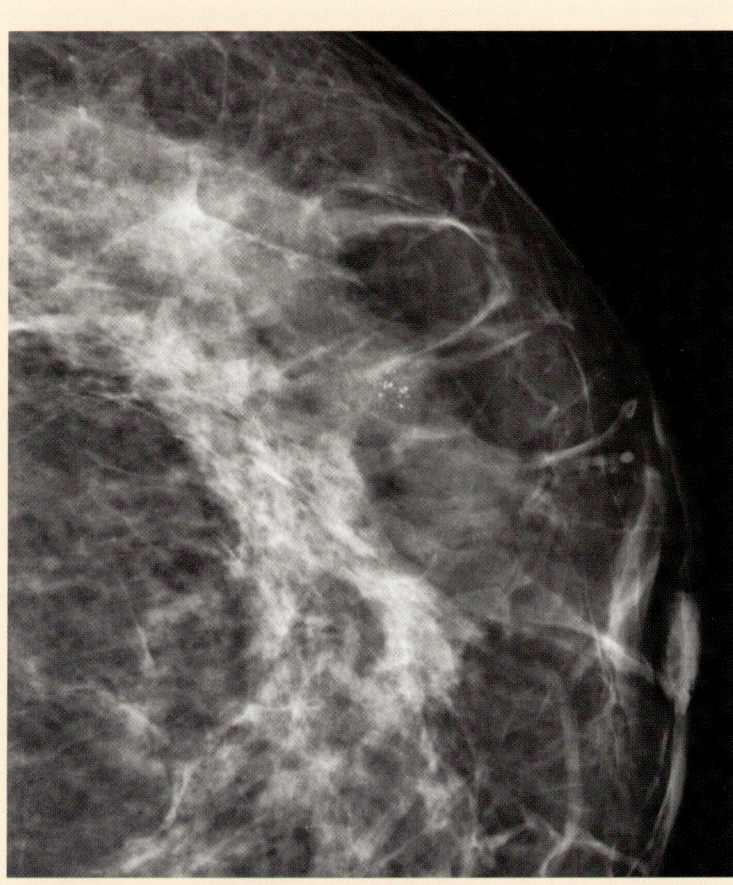

Zoomed left CC view

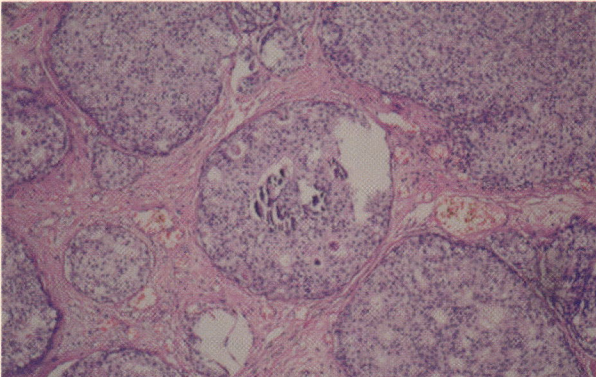

HPE left breast lesion

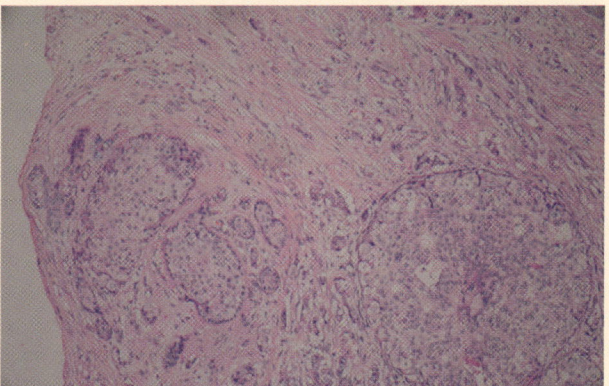

HPE right breast lesion

Key Points

Mammography should always be done for both breasts even in the clinical setting of malignant appearing mass lesion in one breast with no clinical abnormality in the other.

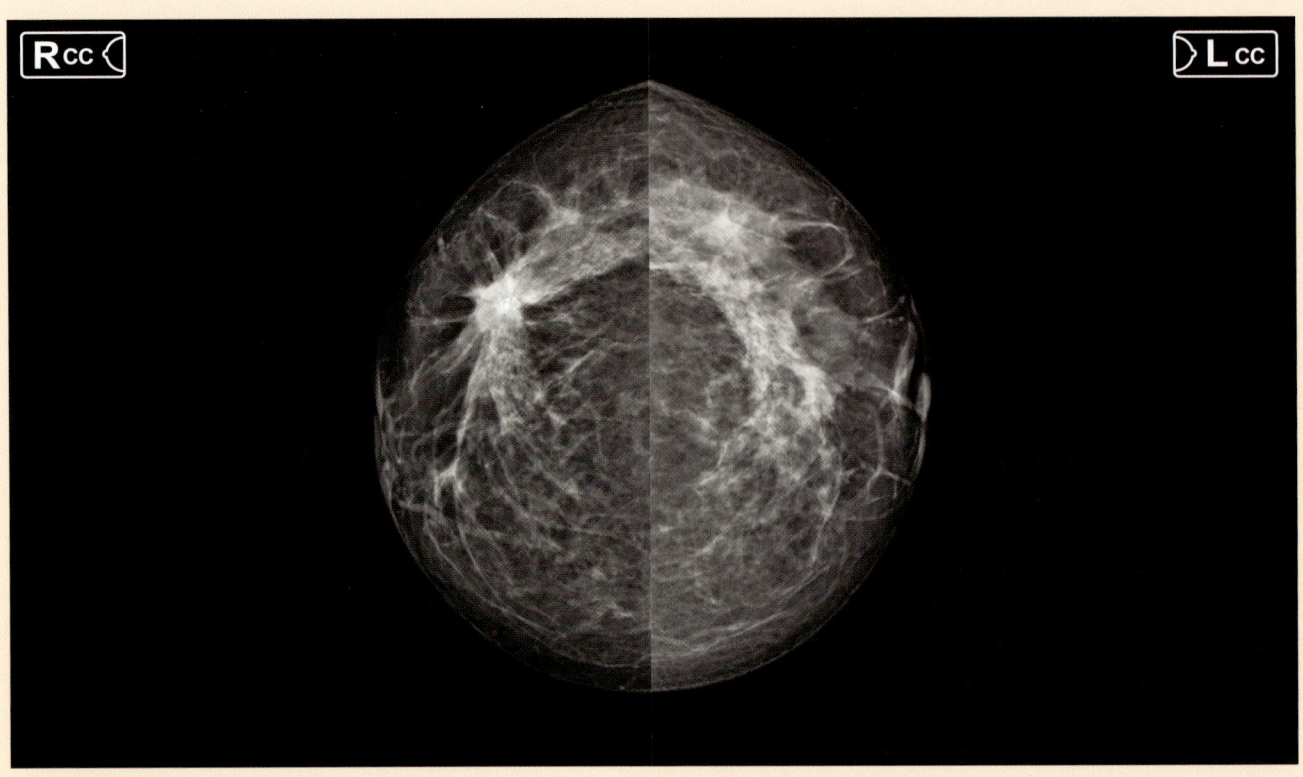

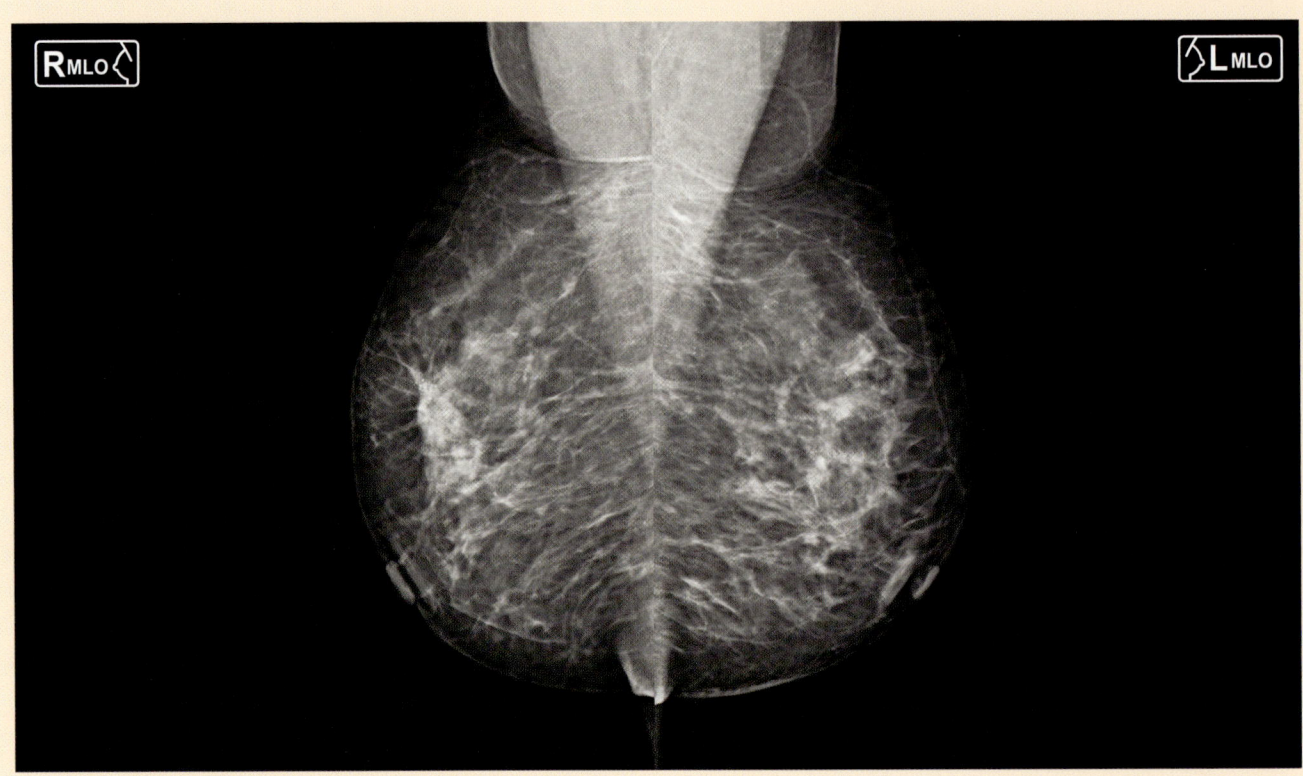

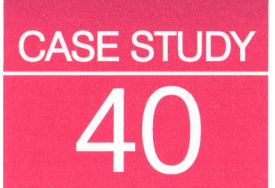

73-year-old lady with palpable lump in left breast

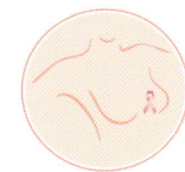

Mammography

ACR Type B density.

A few small nodular lesions with irregular outline in the upper-inner quadrant of left breast arranged in a ductal distribution. No associated architectural distortion/ internal calcification.

Left breast: BIRADS IV. Suggested HPE correlation. USG-guided FNAC from left breast lump positive for malignant cells.

Left MRM HPE: Mucinous carcinoma with foci of DCIS.

FNAC image

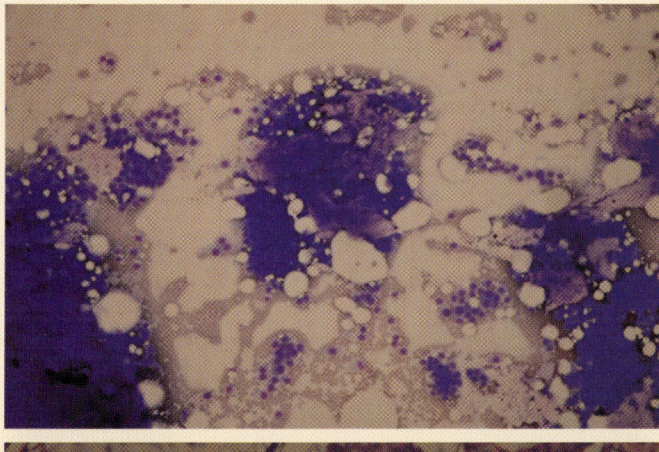

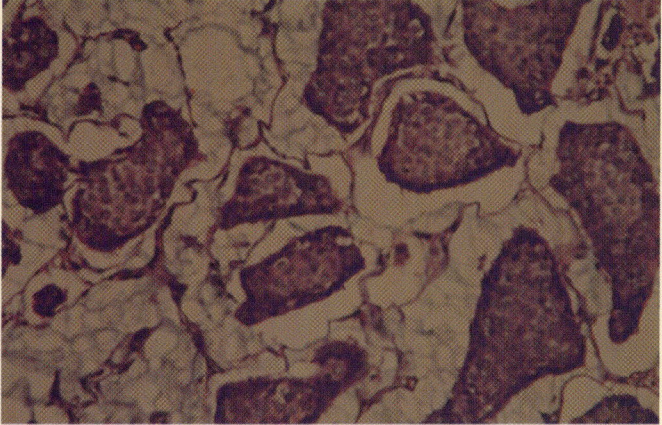

HPE image

Key Points

Clustered soft tissue lesions in segmental/ductal distribution are suspicious of underlying malignancy should be evaluated further by FNAC / biopsy.

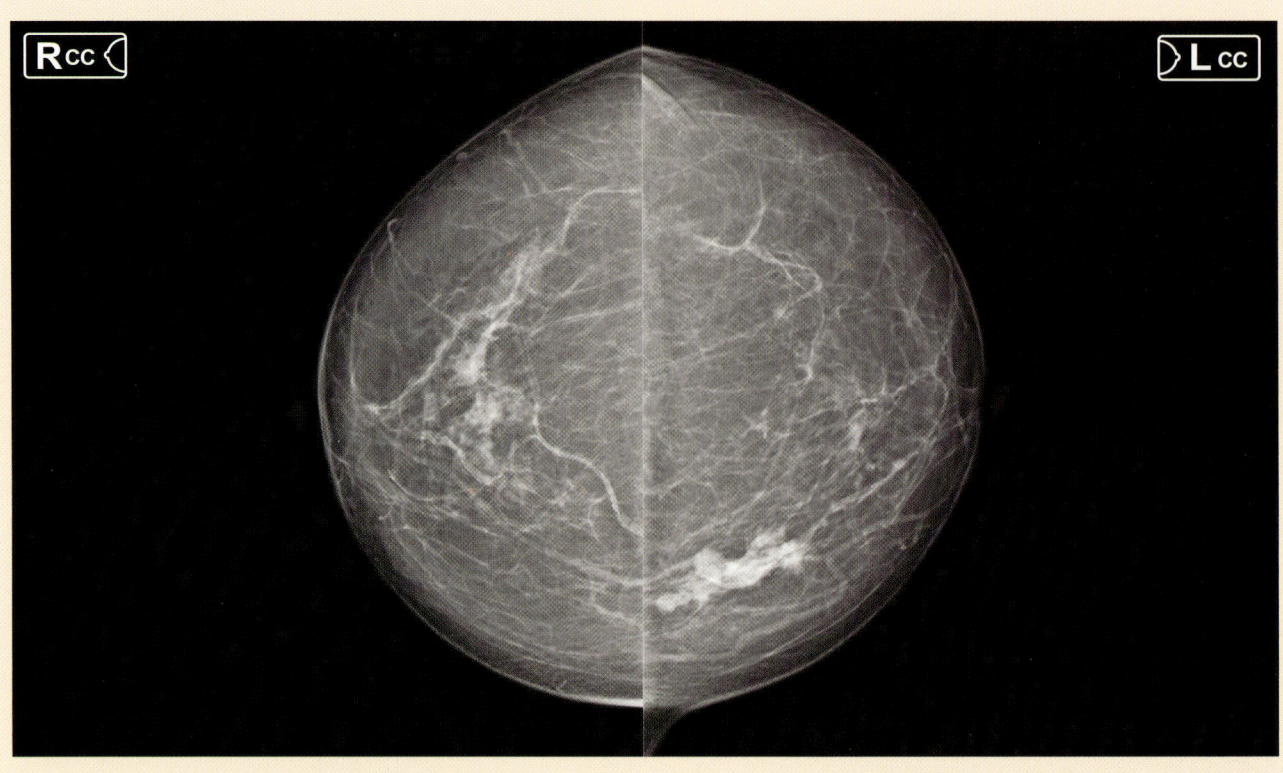

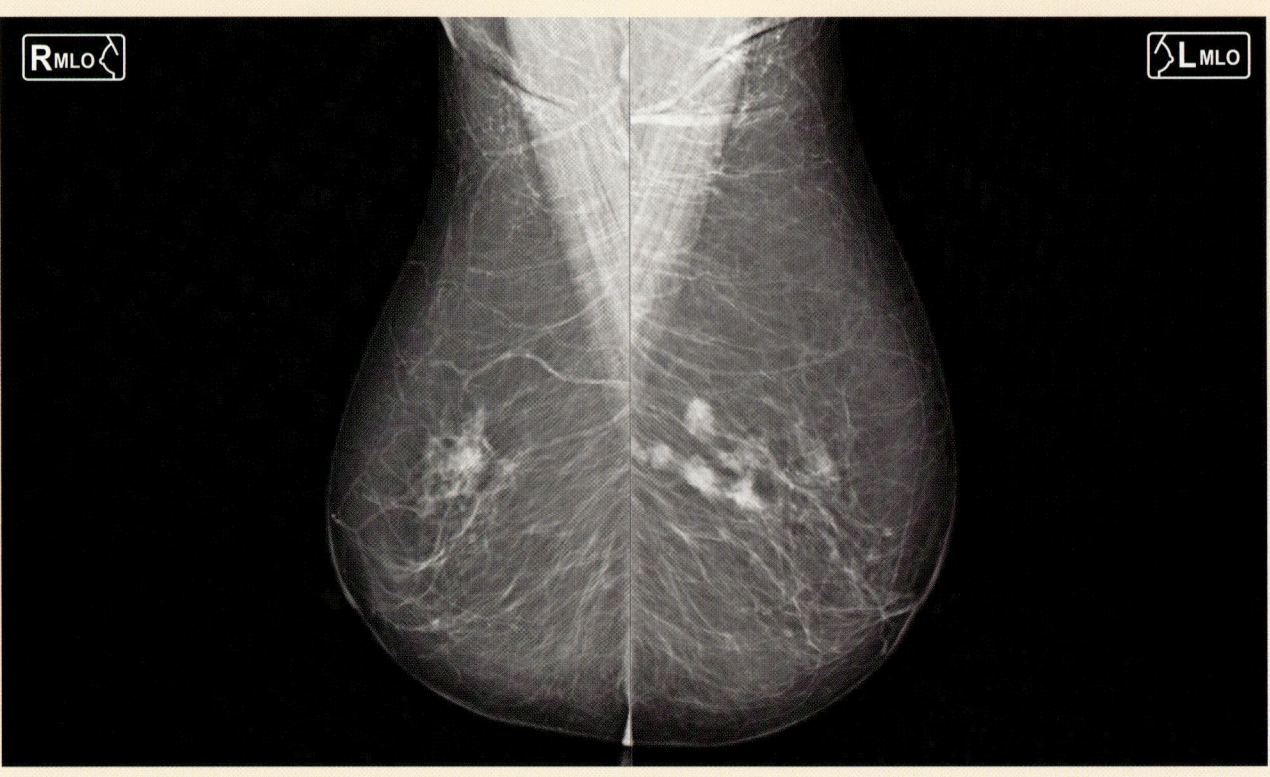

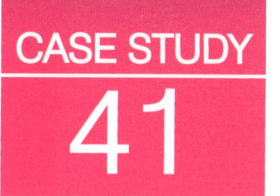

CASE STUDY 41

43-year-old lady presenting with right breast lump

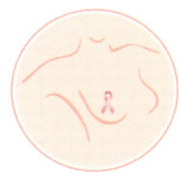

Mammography

ACR Type B density.

Spiculated soft tissue mass lesion in upper-outer quadrant with associated architectural distortion with thickening, puckering of overlying skin.

BIRADS V

Right breast biopsy: Invasive ductal carcinoma.

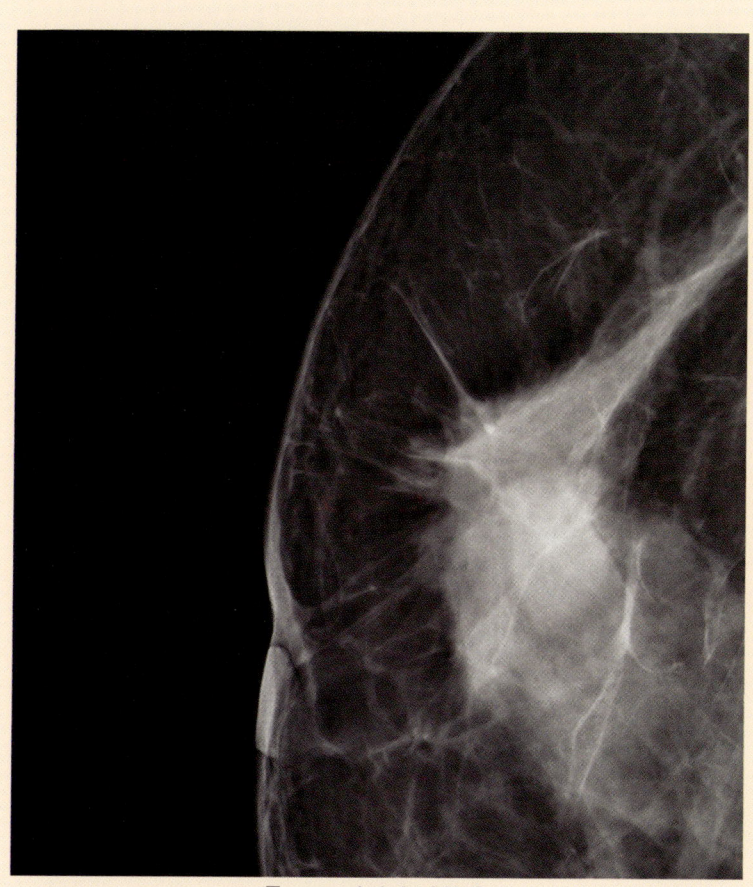

Zoomed right MLO

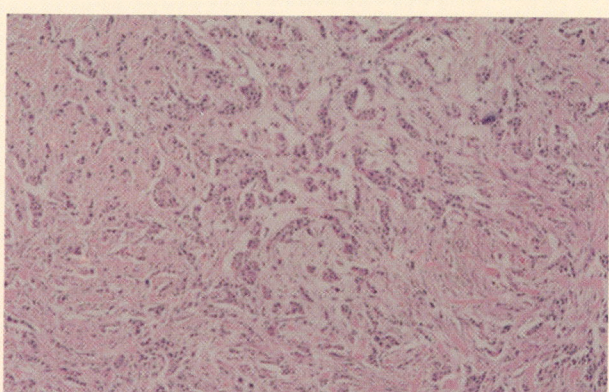

HPE image

Key Points

Secondary signs of underlying mass are focal thickening, puckering of skin and retraction of nipple. These signs are easily identified and should alert the radiologist to look for a mass lesion in the underlying breast parenchyma. The mass in this case is highlighted mainly by the secondary features.

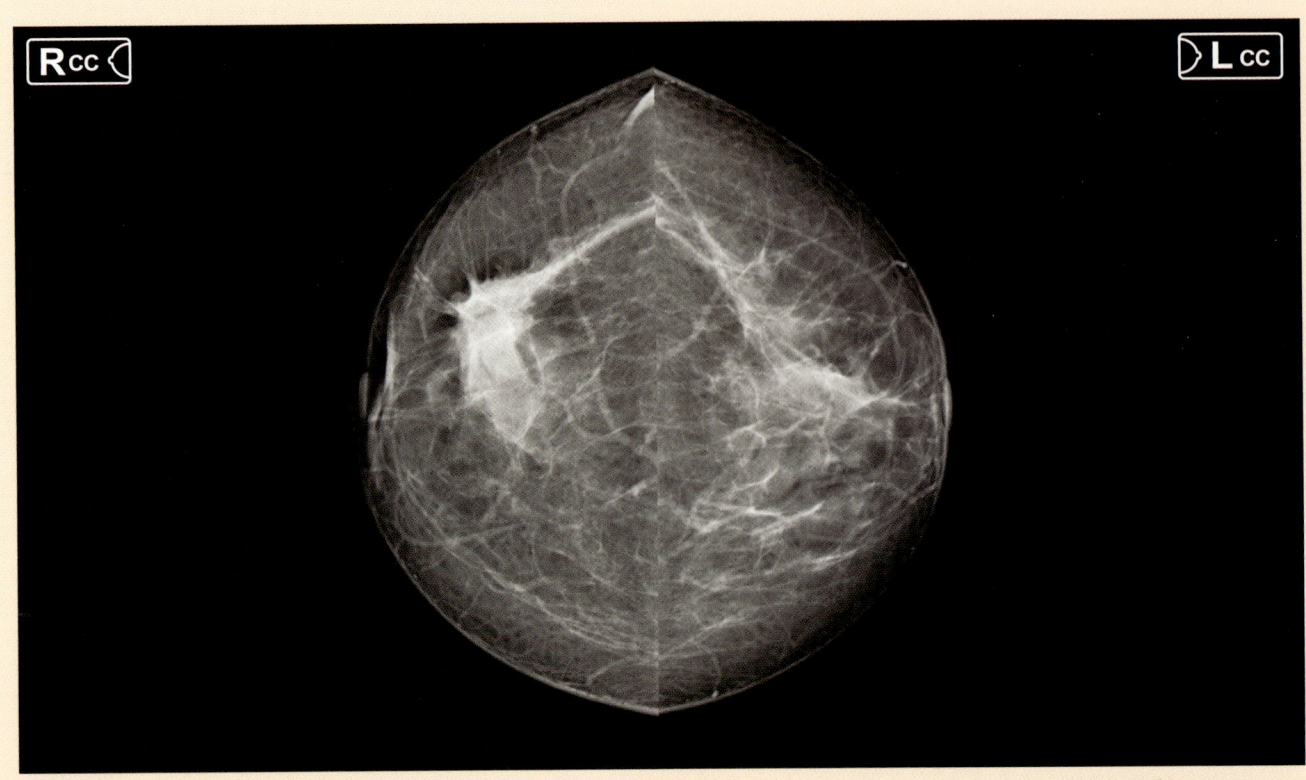

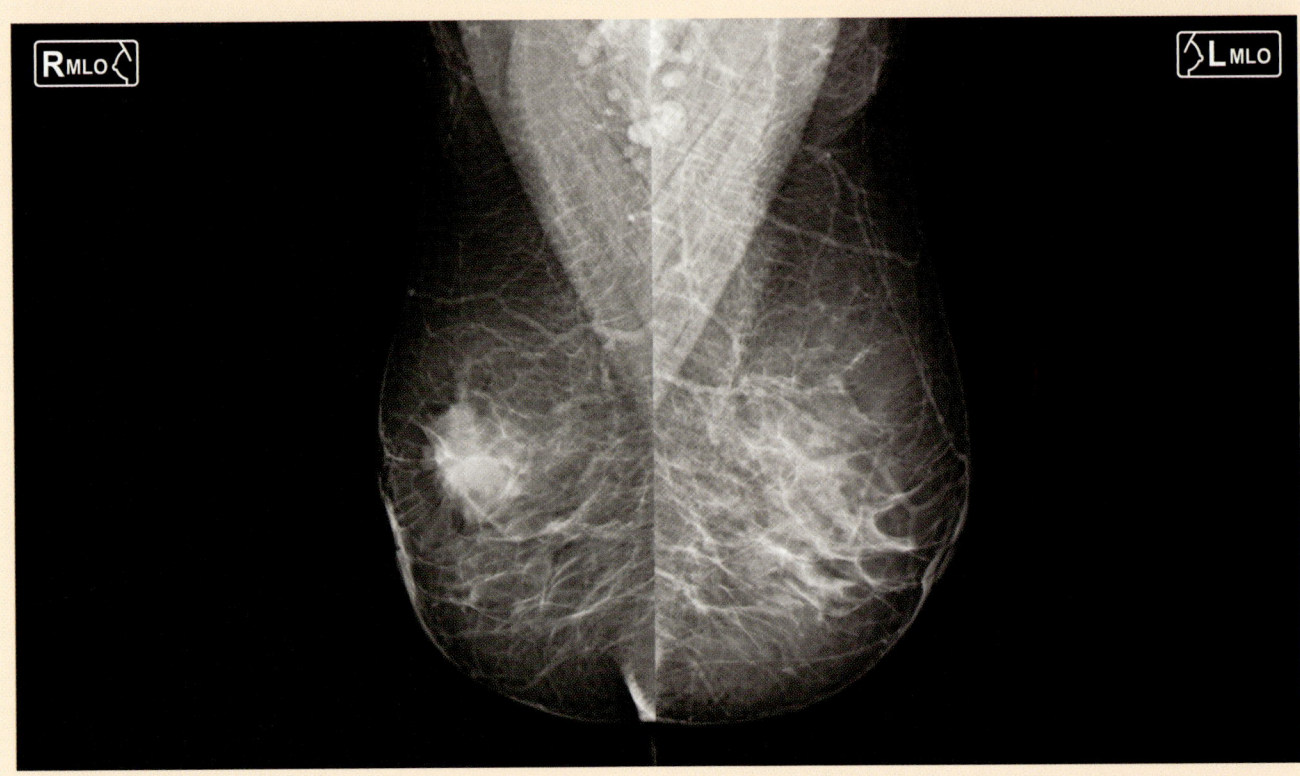

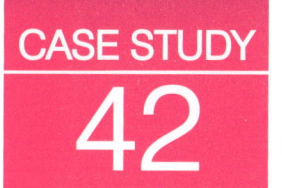
58-year-old lady with left breast lump

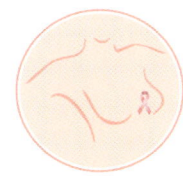

Mammography

ACR Type B density.

Large soft tissue mass lesion of 6 x 4 cm size in upper-outer quadrant of left breast. The lesion shows a differentially denser soft tissue component with irregular outline and internal micro-, macro-calcifications with relatively less dense component showing a smooth margin. Enlarged left axillary node seen. Left breast BIRADS V.

USG shows a solid cystic lesion with smooth outline of the cystic component and irregular outline of a portion of the solid component.

Left breast lesion HPE: Invasive carcinoma with metaplastic features.

Left breast FNAC: Features favouring hight grade DCIS.

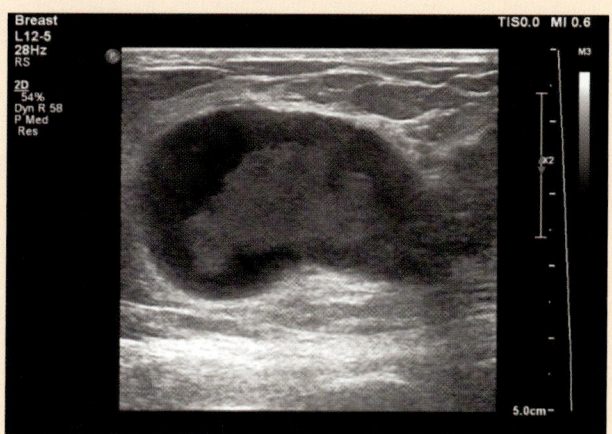

USG image of left breast lesion

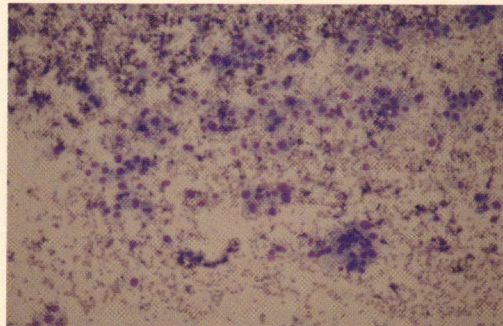

FNAC image

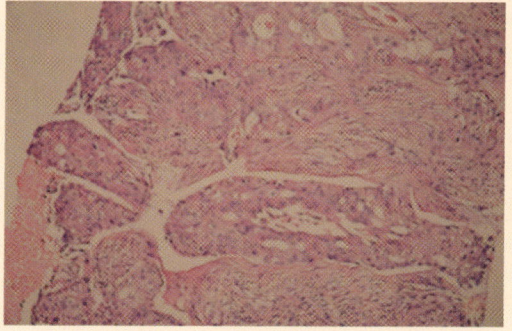

HPE image

Key Points

Solid cystic lesions can have differential densities of the solid and cystic components, as in this case. The margin of the denser solid component should be critically evaluated for any irregularity.

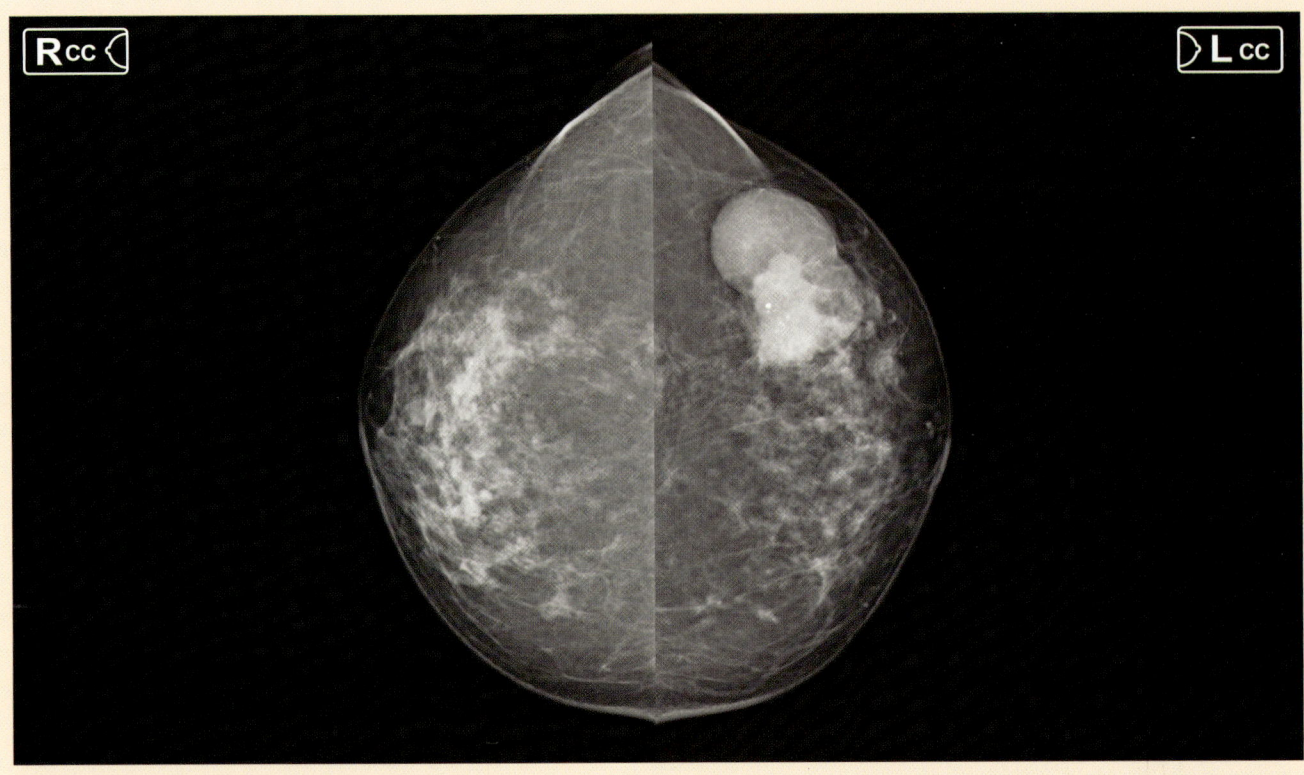

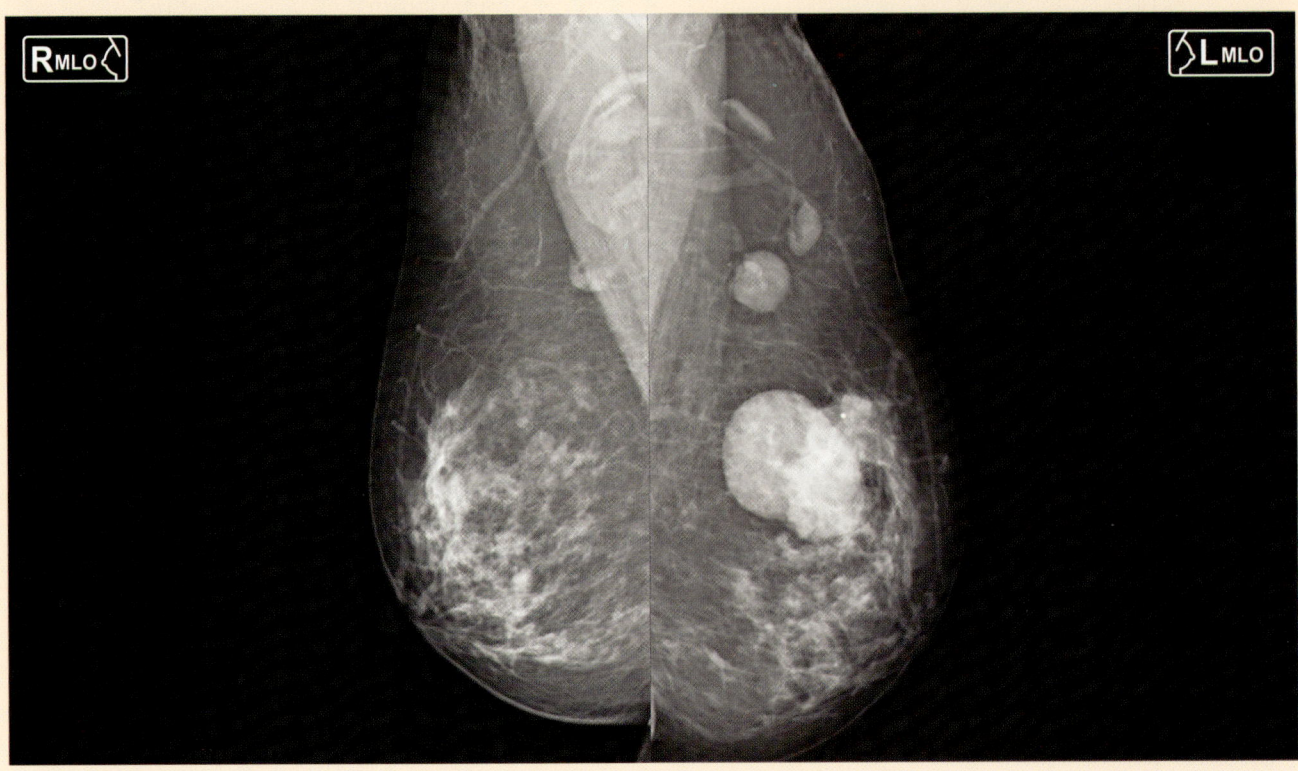

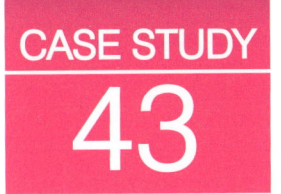

CASE STUDY 43

42-year-old lady presenting with lump in right breast

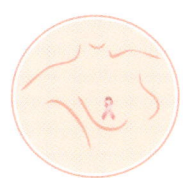

Mammography

Shows extremely dense parenchyma (ACR type D)

Rounded dense soft tissue lesion with smooth outline in the region of axillary tail of right breast.

BIRADS IV

USG-guided FNAC: Positive for malignant cells.

MRM: Invasive mammary carcinoma.

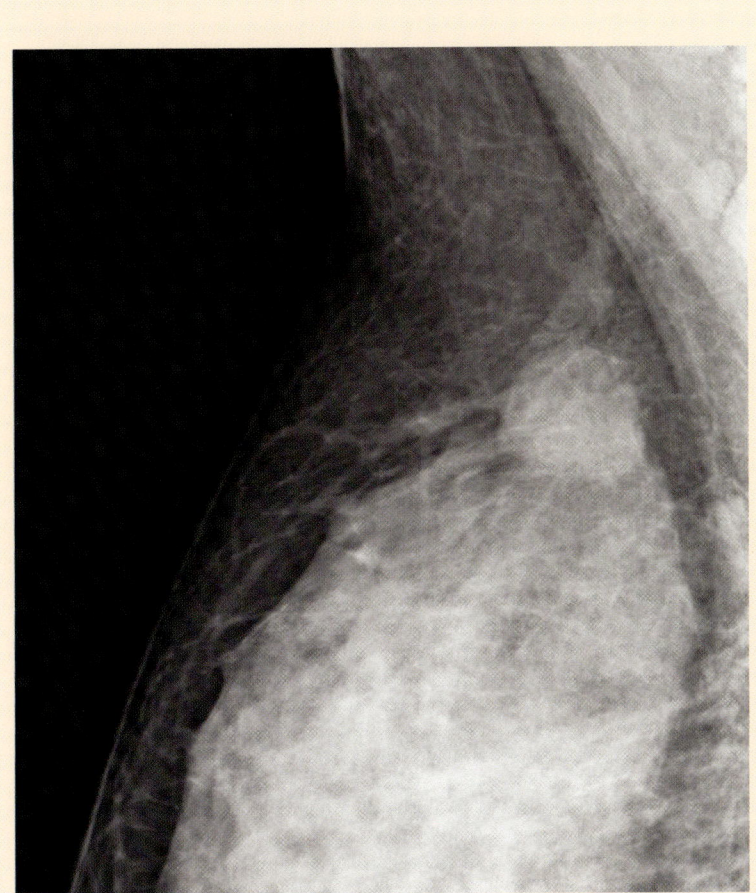

Zoomed right MLO

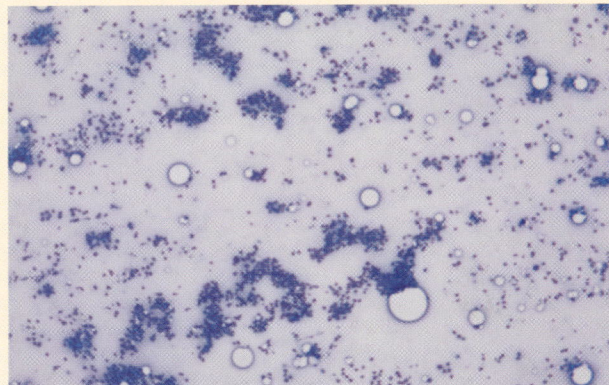

FNAC image

Key Points

It is difficult to pick focal soft tissue lesions in the background of extremely dense breast parenchyma. Clinical findings should always be noted before evaluation of mammography. In case mammography findings do not explain the clinical findings, a BIRADS 0 should be given and further imaging done with USG/MRI. Axillary lesions are often not seen in the CC view as in this case.

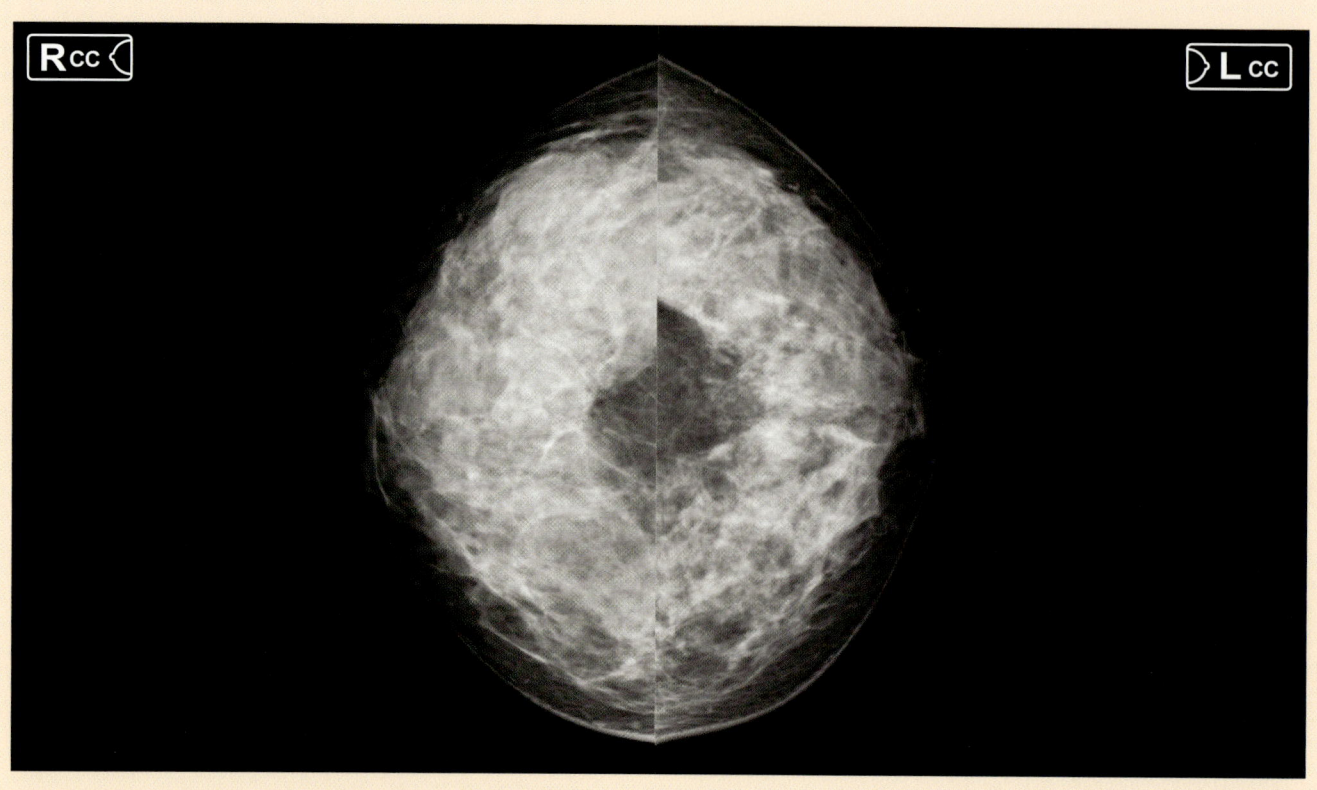

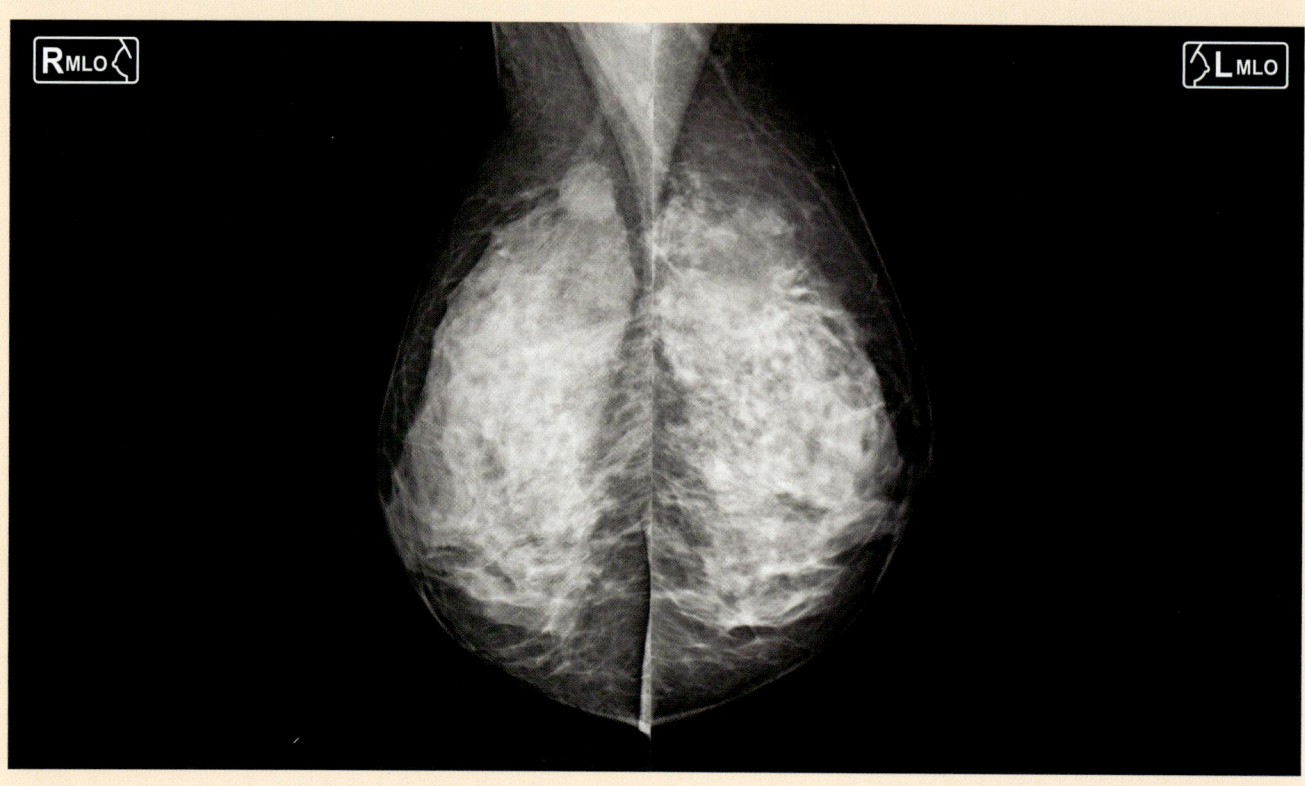

55-year-old lady presenting with right axillary mass

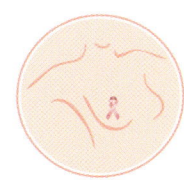

Mammography

Bilateral breasts show ACR Type B density.

Right breast shows multiple egg shell type benign macrocalcifications.

Small rounded soft tissue with lucent halo is seen projected in upper-inner quadrant consistent with known mole in this region.

No definite suspicious focal mass/architectural distortion/clustered microcalcification seen on either side.

Multiple enlarged, dense right axillary nodes with no discernible hilar lucency.

BIRADS 0

Suggested MRI breast with FNAC of right axillary nodes.

Right axillary node FNAC revealed poorly differentiated carcinoma.

Patient opted for PET-CT instead of MRI breast.

PET-CT revealed a small nodular soft tissue lesion with FDG uptake in the upper quadrant of right breast with enlarged hypermetabolic nodes.

MRM HPE: Revealed a firm gray white tumor in upper quadrant of right breast, measuring 15 × 13 × 10 mm. Microscopy revealed invasive carcinoma.

PET-CT images

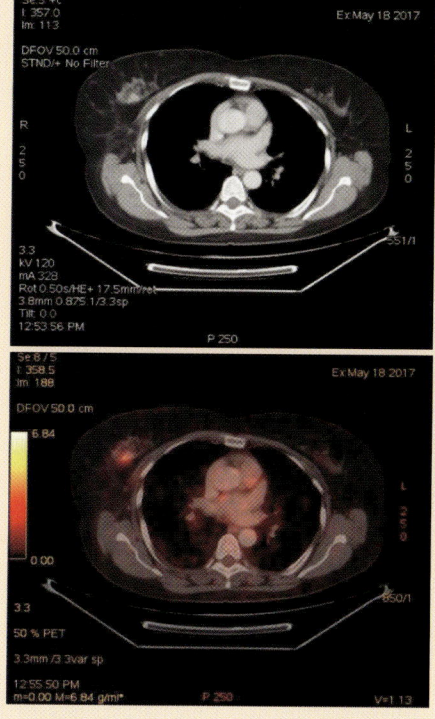

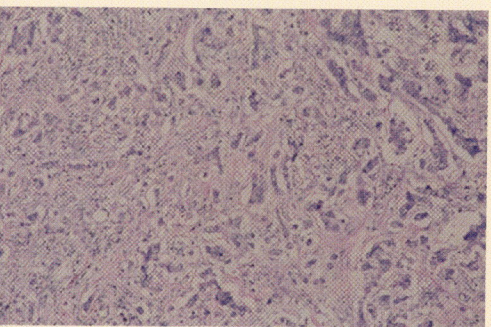

MRM HPE image

Key Points

All mammary carcinomas are not seen on mammography. Further evaluation by USG/MRI needs to be done in the clinical setting of high suspicion of breast primary. Abnormal axillary nodes should be subjected to FNA/biopsy.

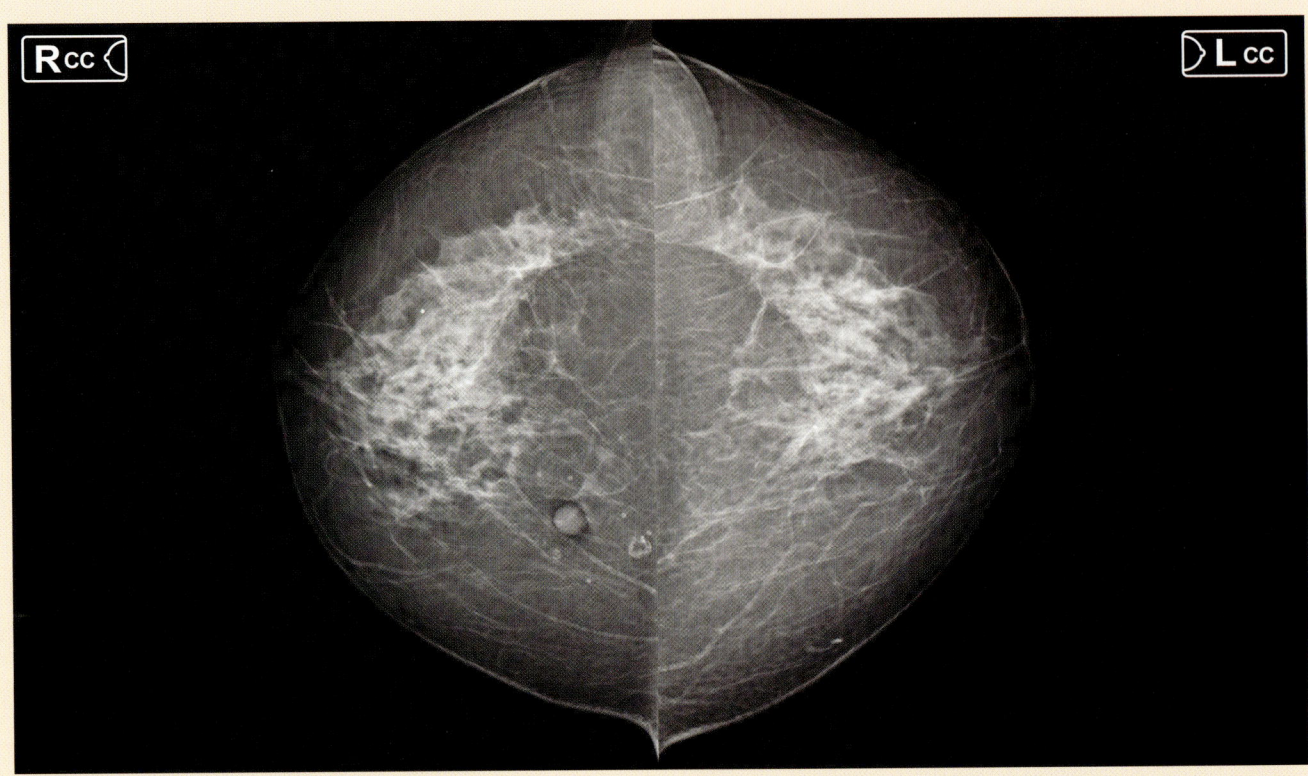

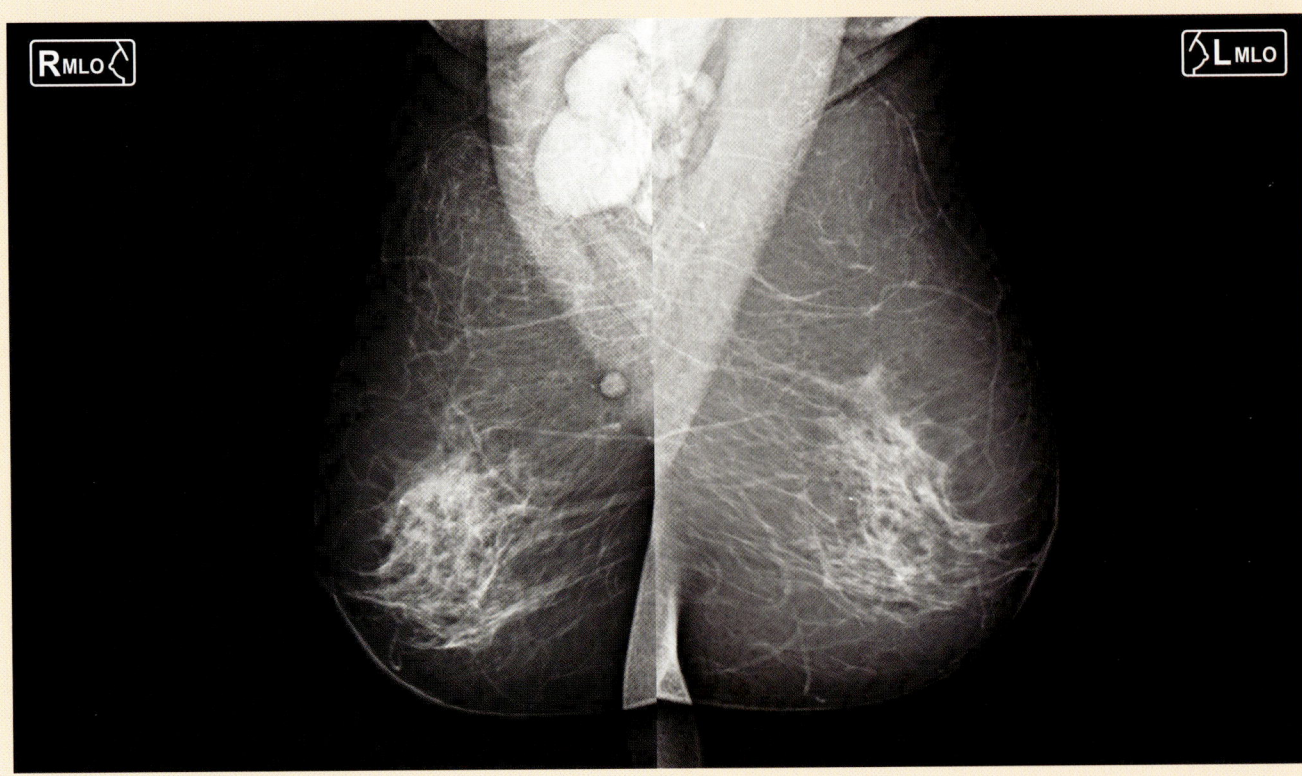

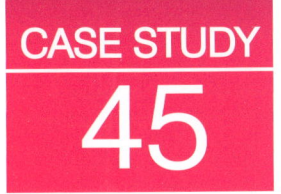

51-year-old lady presenting with lump in left breast

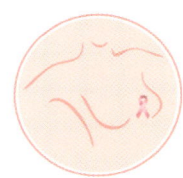

Mammography

ACR Type B density.

Two adjacent placed rounded soft tissue nodular lesions in upper-inner quadrant, showing irregular margins.

BIRADS IVc/ V

HPE: Invasive mammary carcinoma

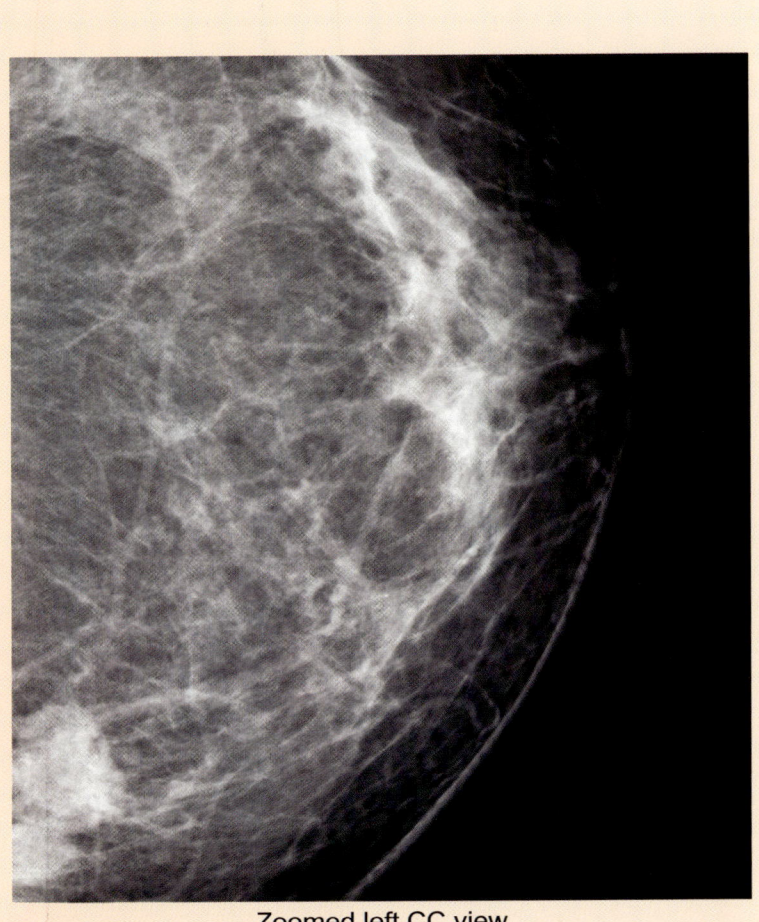

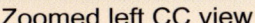

Zoomed left CC view

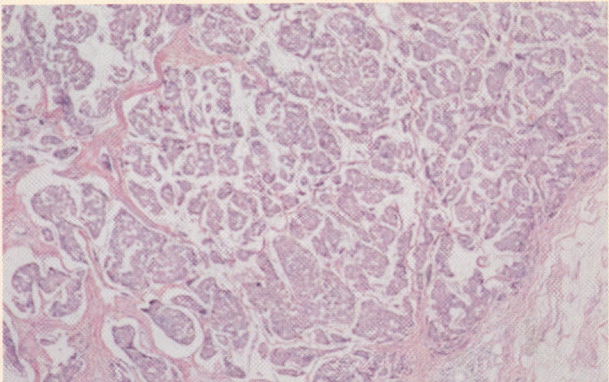

HPE image

Key Points

Meticulous positioning is essential to pick lesions close to the chest wall as in this case. Clinical history and brief examination of the patient by the technologist, before performing mammography, is very helpful.

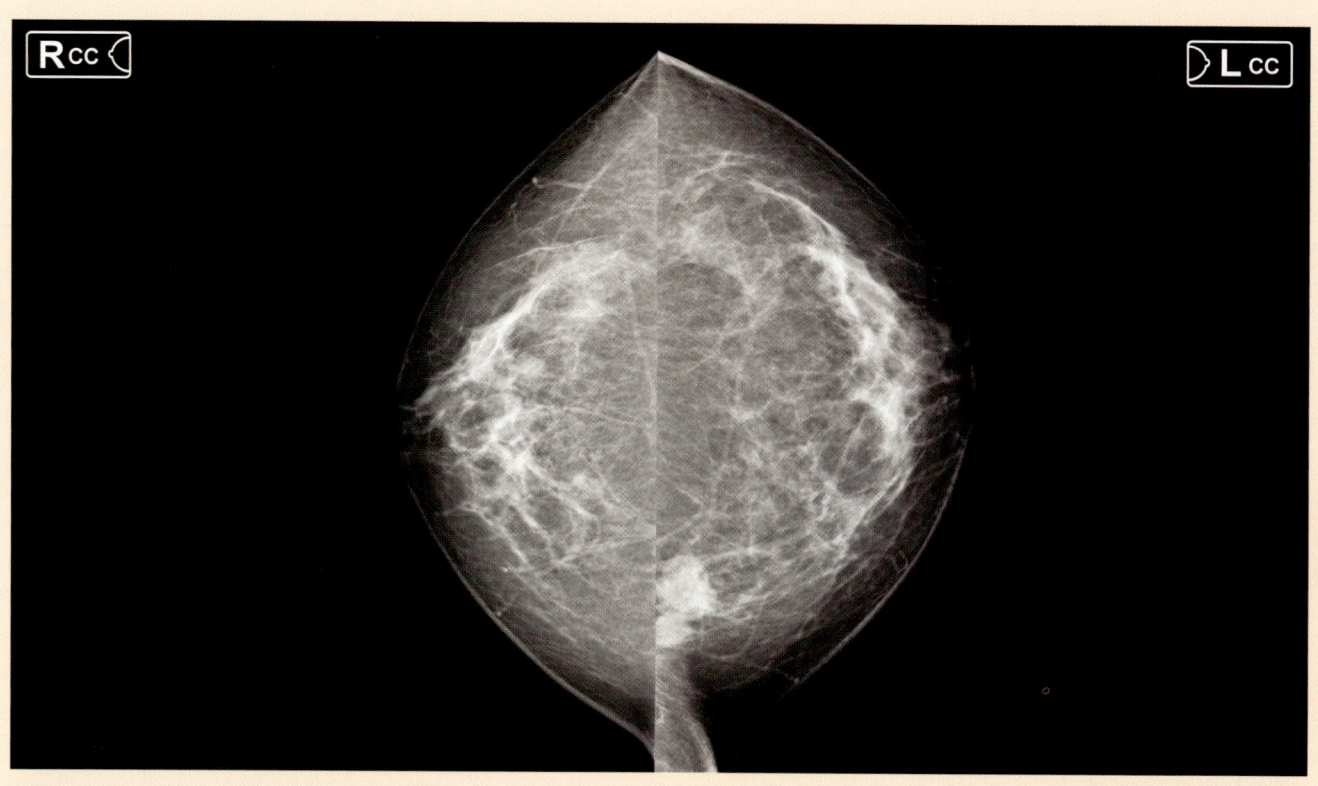

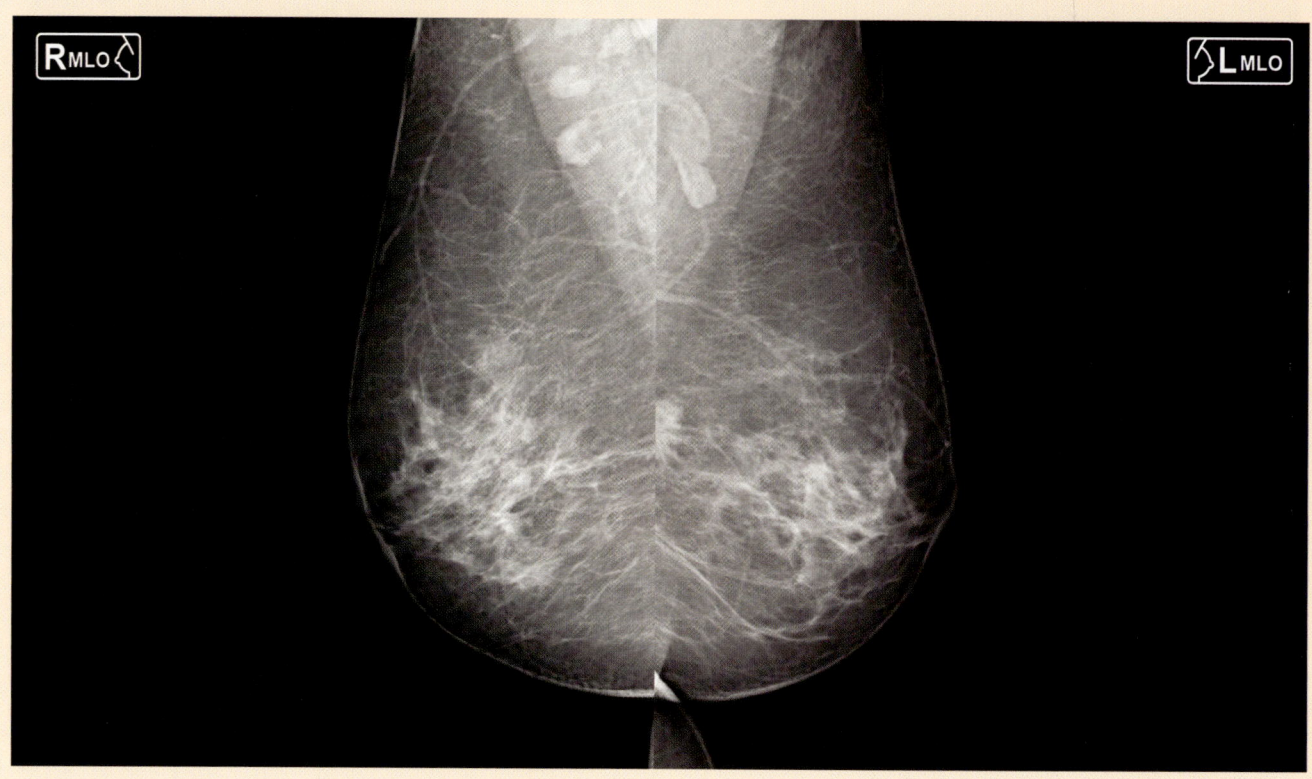

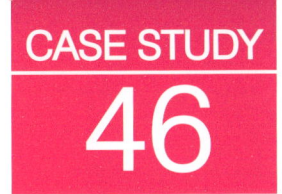

70-year-old lady for screening

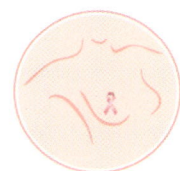

Mammography

ACR Type A density.

Soft tissue lesion with microlobulations and irregularity of outline in outer quadrant of left breast.

BIRADS V

USG-guided FNAC: Positive for malignancy.

Left breast MRM: Mucinous carcinoma.

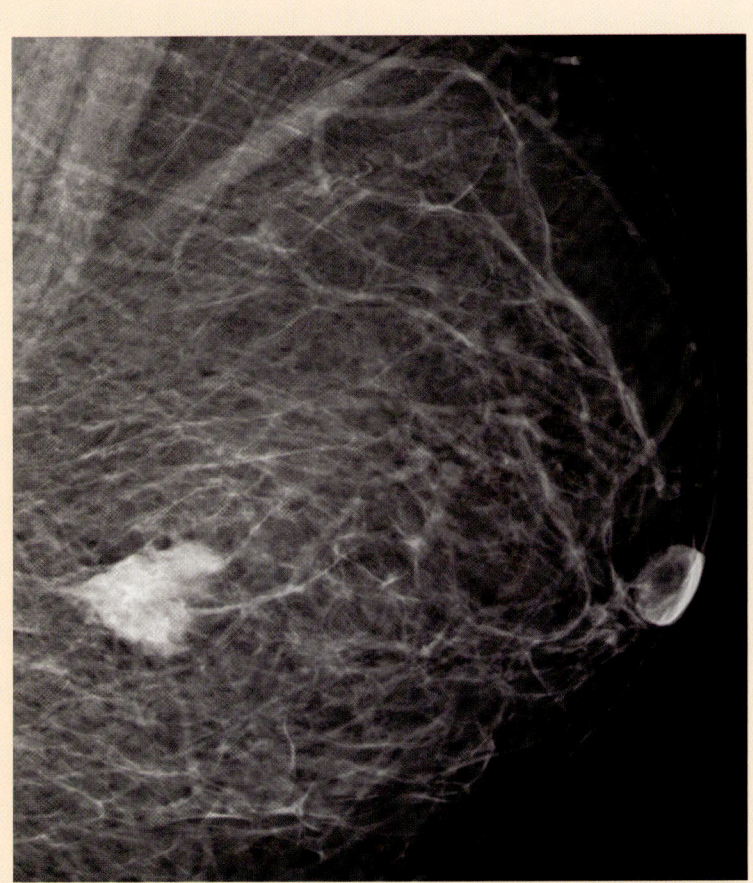

Zoomed left MLO image

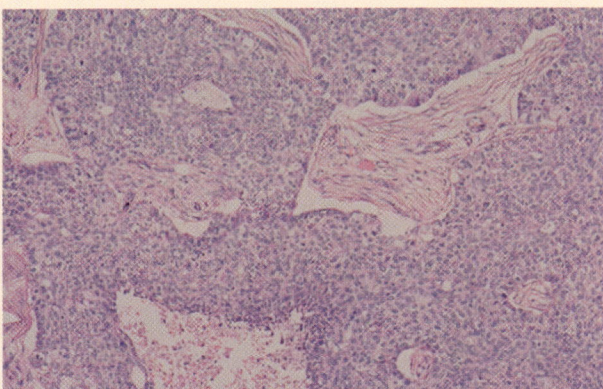

MRM HPE image

Key Points

Small mass lesions are most easily picked up in ACR Type A density breasts.

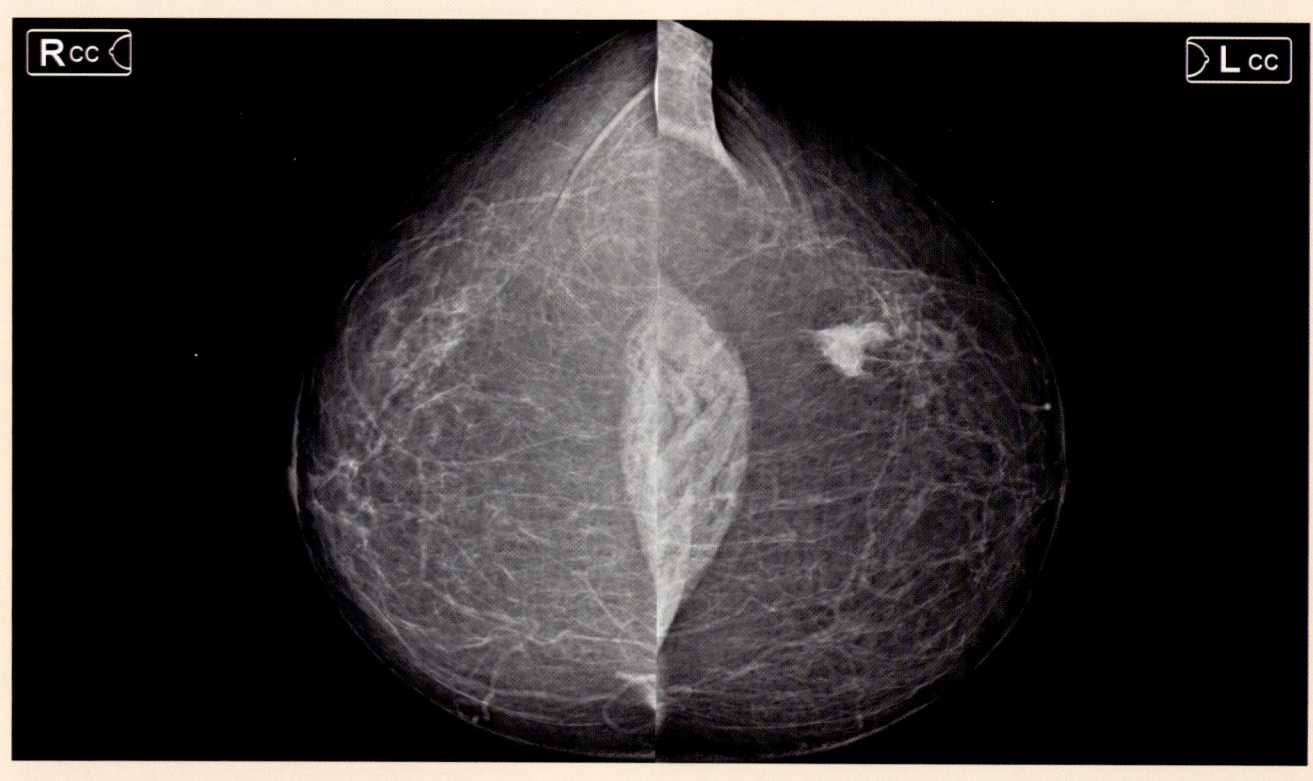

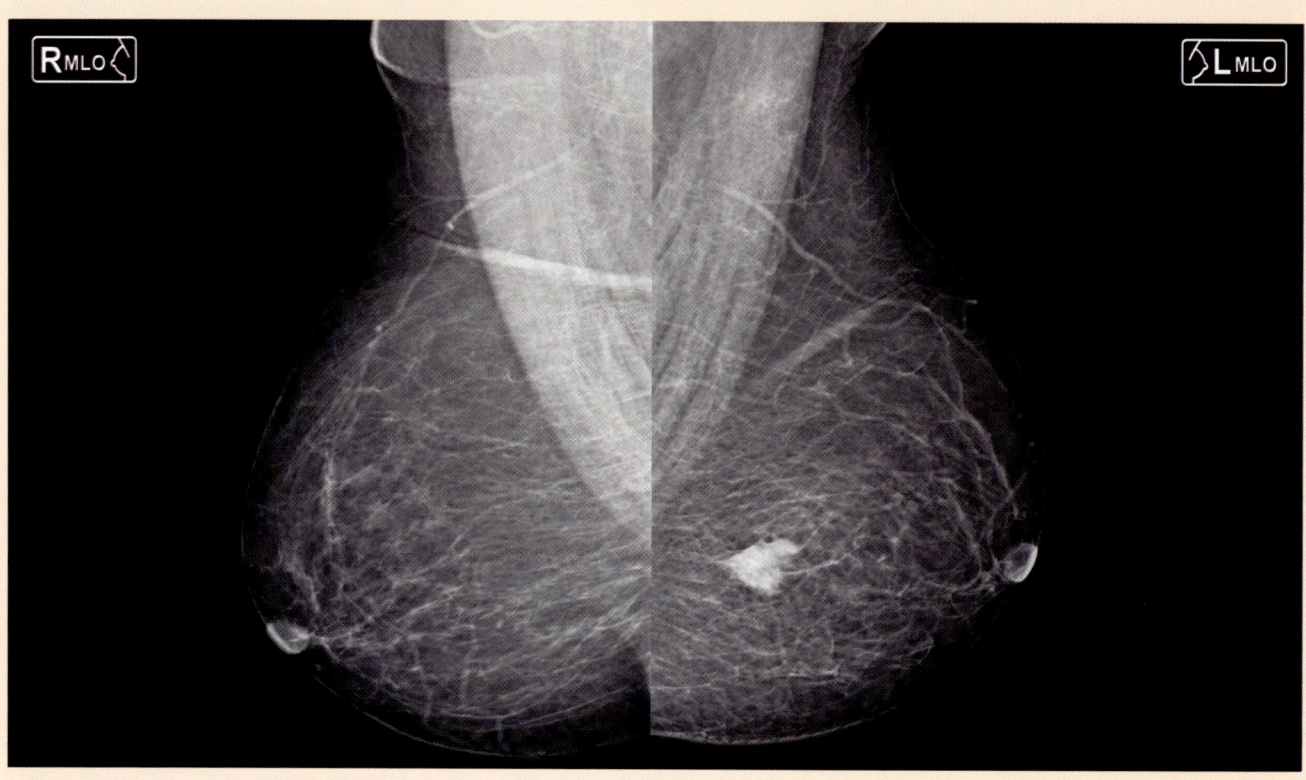

70-year-old female presenting with lump in left breast

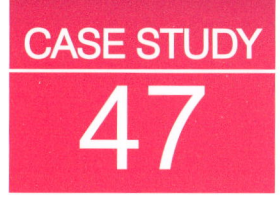
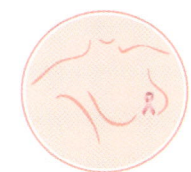

Mammography

ACR Type A density.

Clasical soft tissue lesion with spiculated outline in upper outer quadrant of left breast.

BIRADS V

HPE : Invasive carcinoma

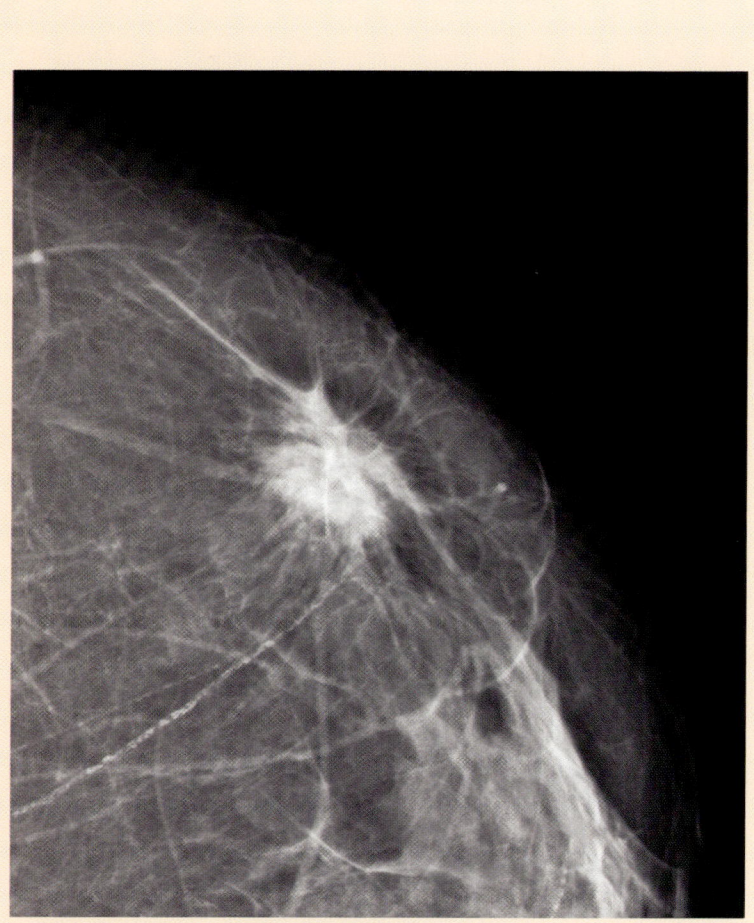

Zoomed left CC view

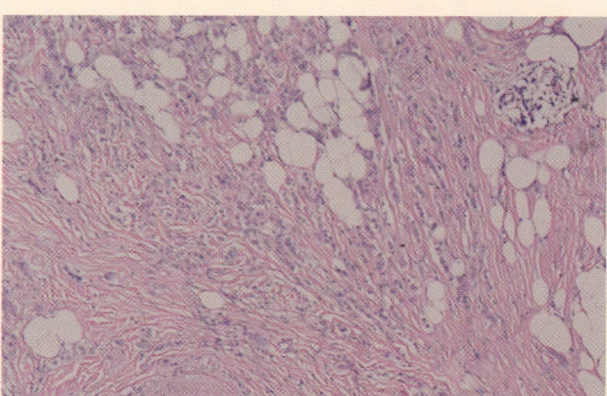

HPE image

Key Points

Soft tissue mass with spiculated outline and architectural distortion in an old lady is typical of a malignant lesion.

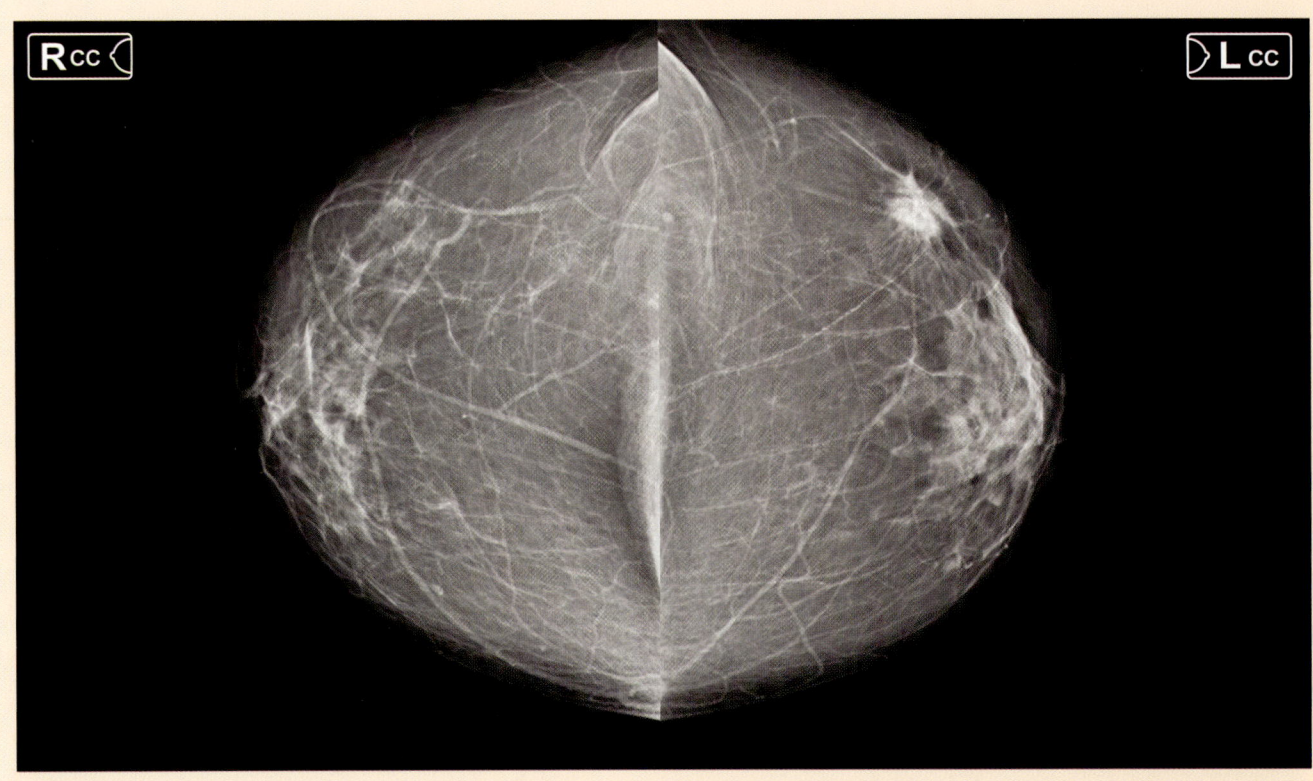

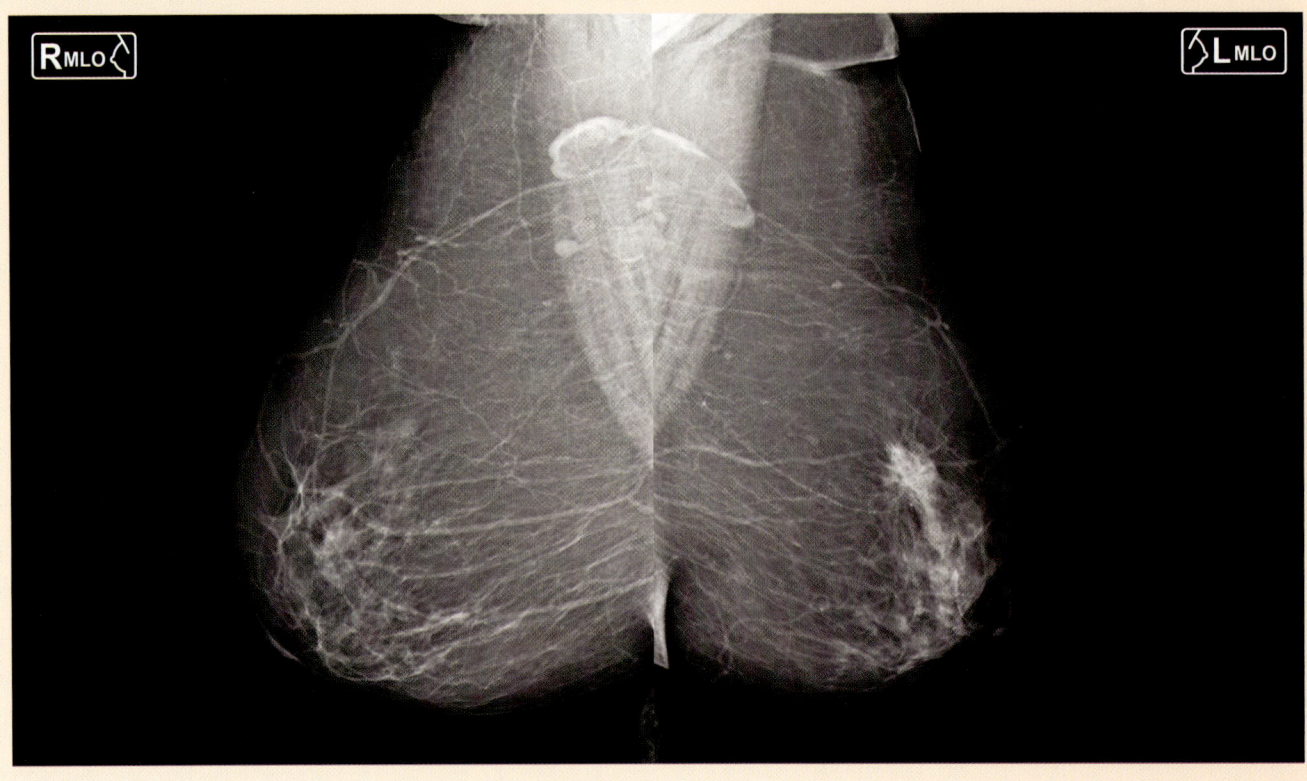

47-year-old lady presenting with right breast lump

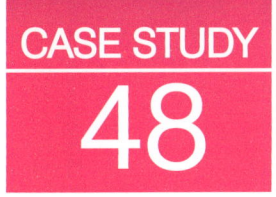
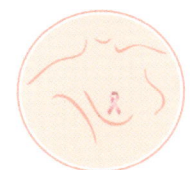

Mammography

ACR Type C density.

Right breast shows a 3 cm lobulated soft tissue lesion with irregular margins.

BIRADS V

USG-guided FNAC: Positive for malignant cells.

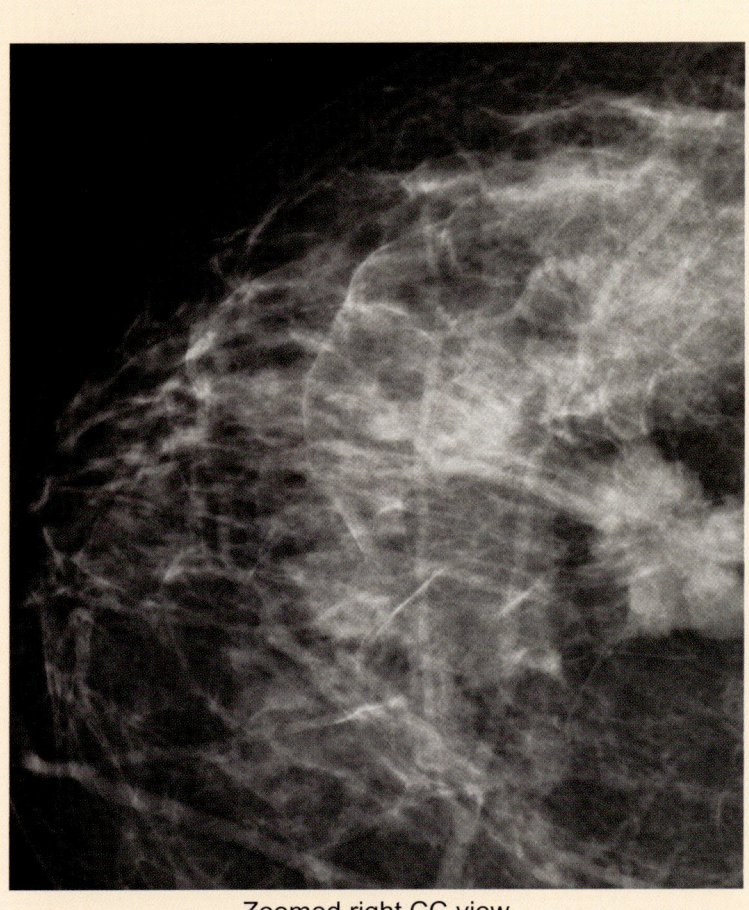

Zoomed right CC view

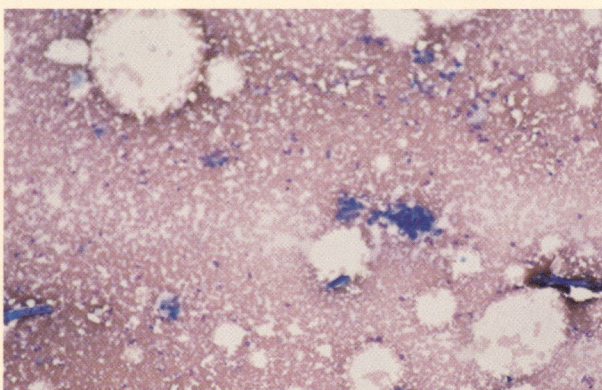

FNAC image

Key Points

Retromammary and retroareolar regions are the review areas and special attention should be given to these areas while evaluating mammography images.

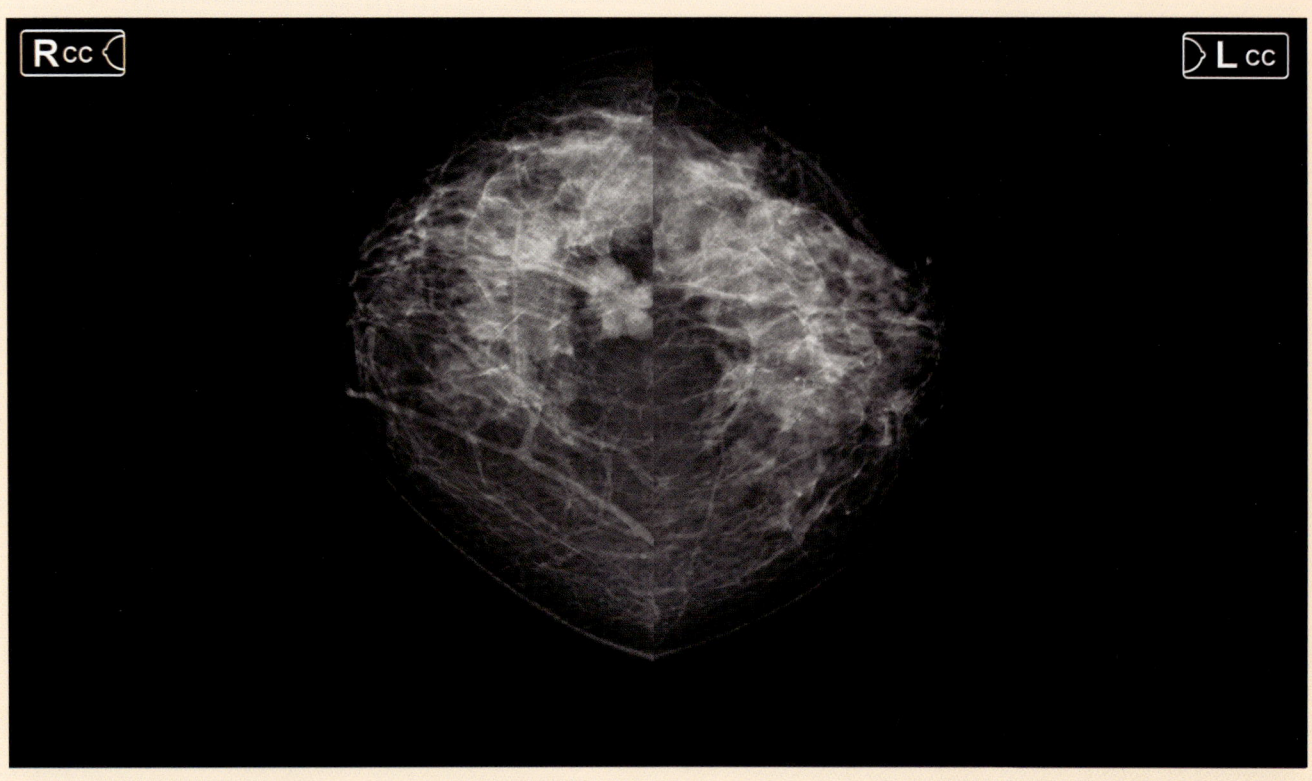

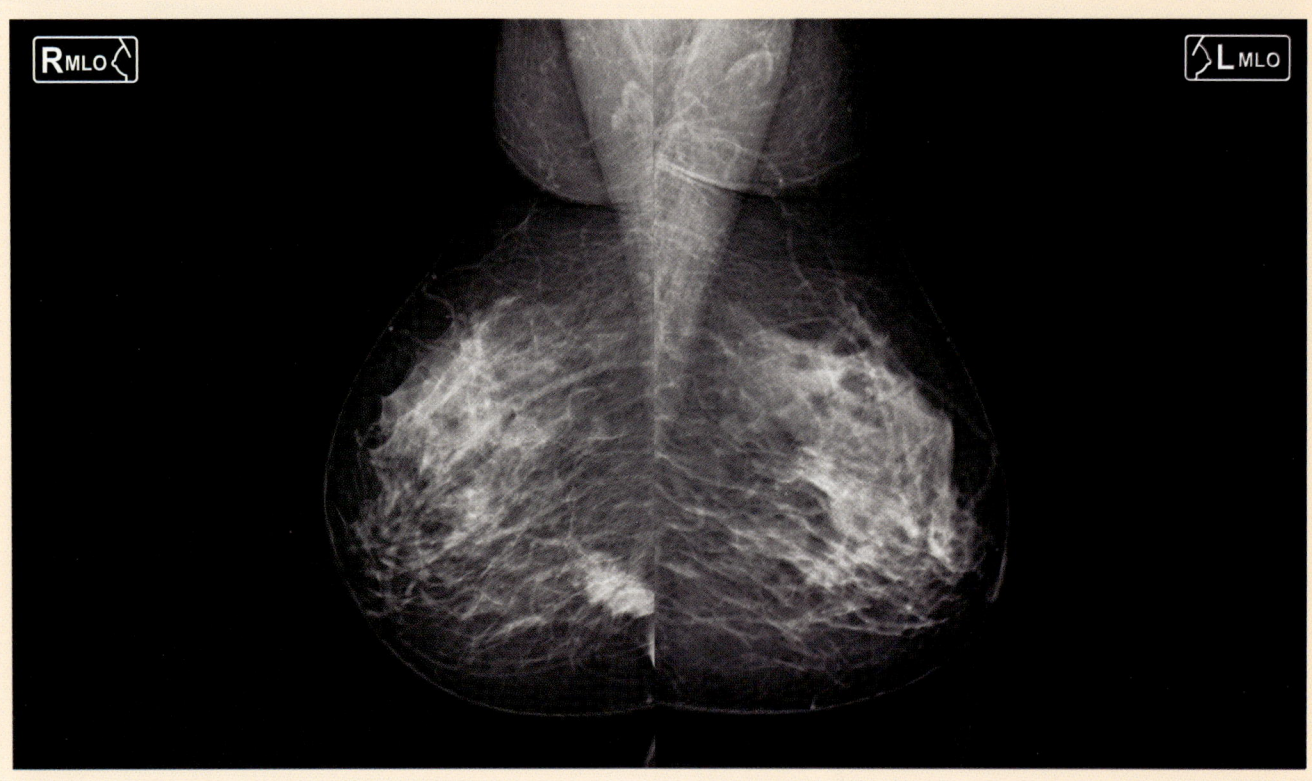

72-year-old female presenting with left breast lump

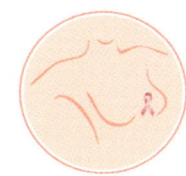

Mammography

Soft tissue mass with poorly defined margins with extensive internal micro-, macro-calcifications in outer quadrant of left breast with associated architectural distortion, thickening, retraction of overlying skin, nipple.

Rounded suspicious node in the left axilla.

BIRADS V

USG-guided biopsy: Invasive carcinoma.

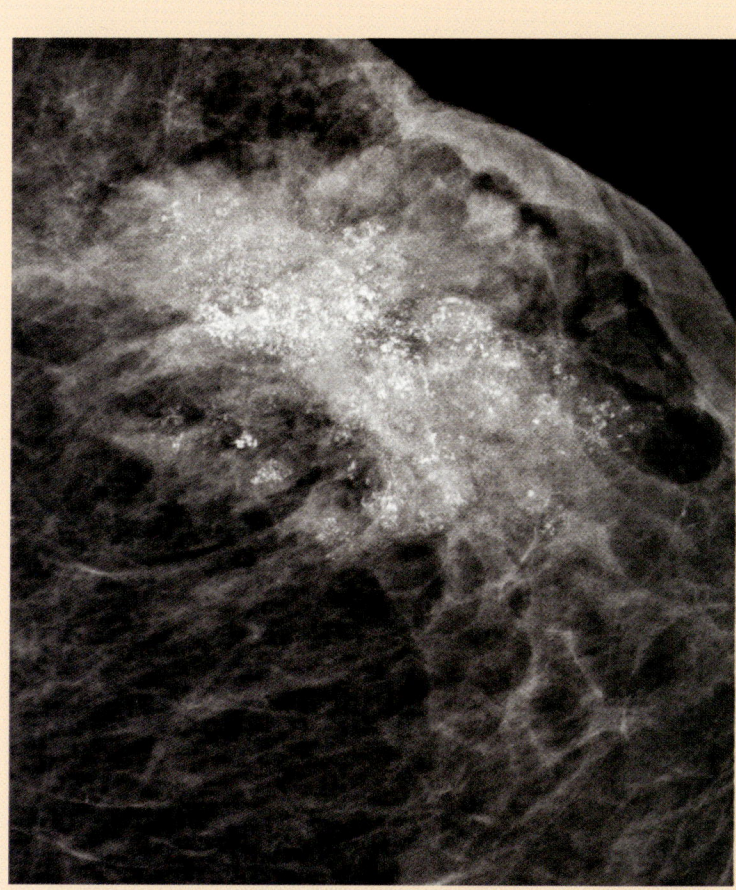

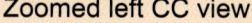

Zoomed left CC view

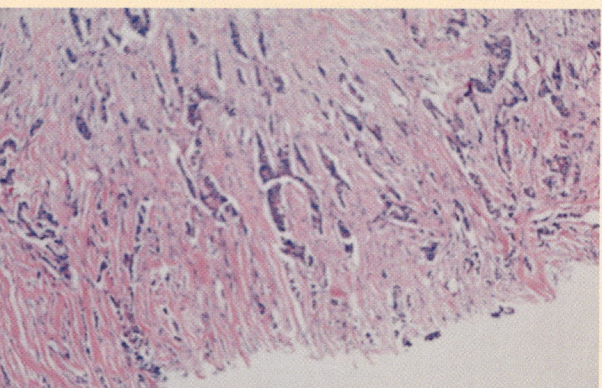

HPE image

Key Points

Amorphous, pleomorphic microcalcifications in regional/segmental/ductal distribution or branching pattern are suspicious for malignancy even in the absence of associated mass. New appearance of clustered pleomorphic microcalcifications are also suspicious.

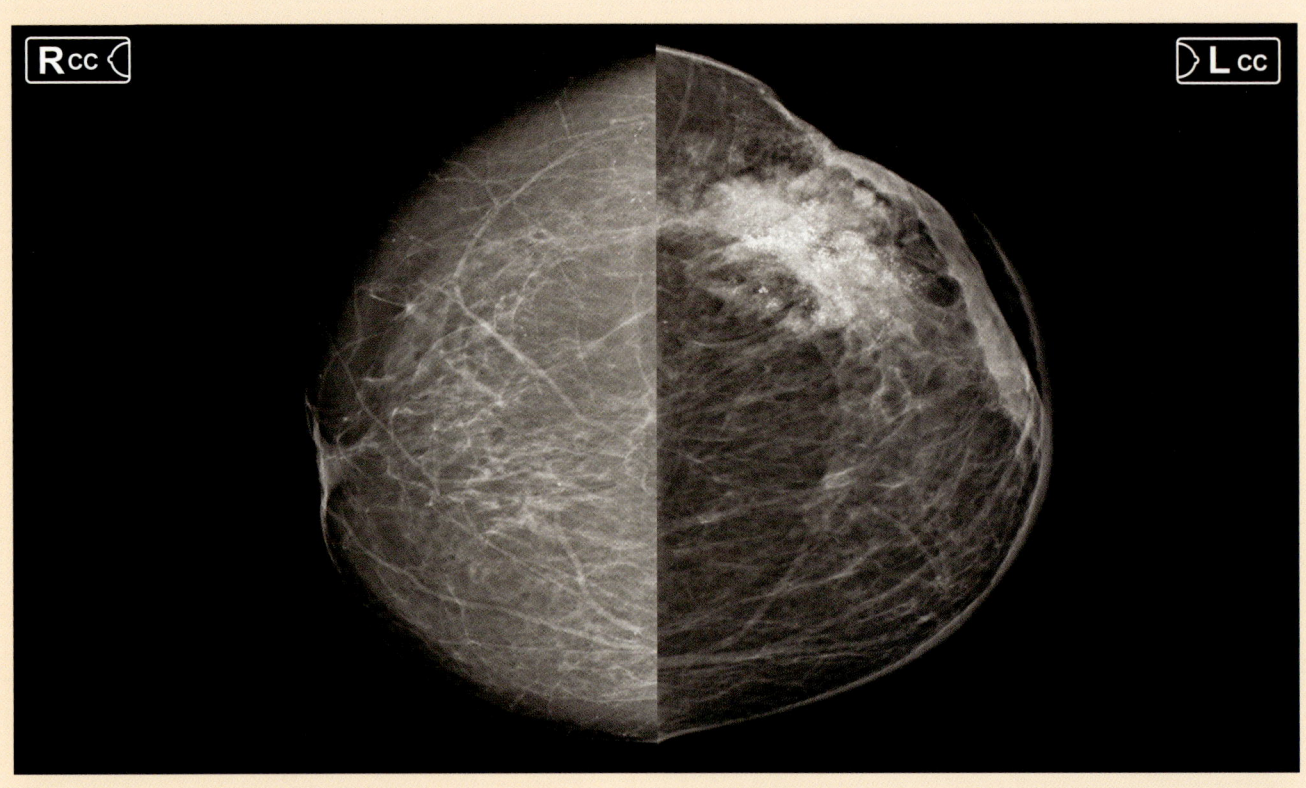

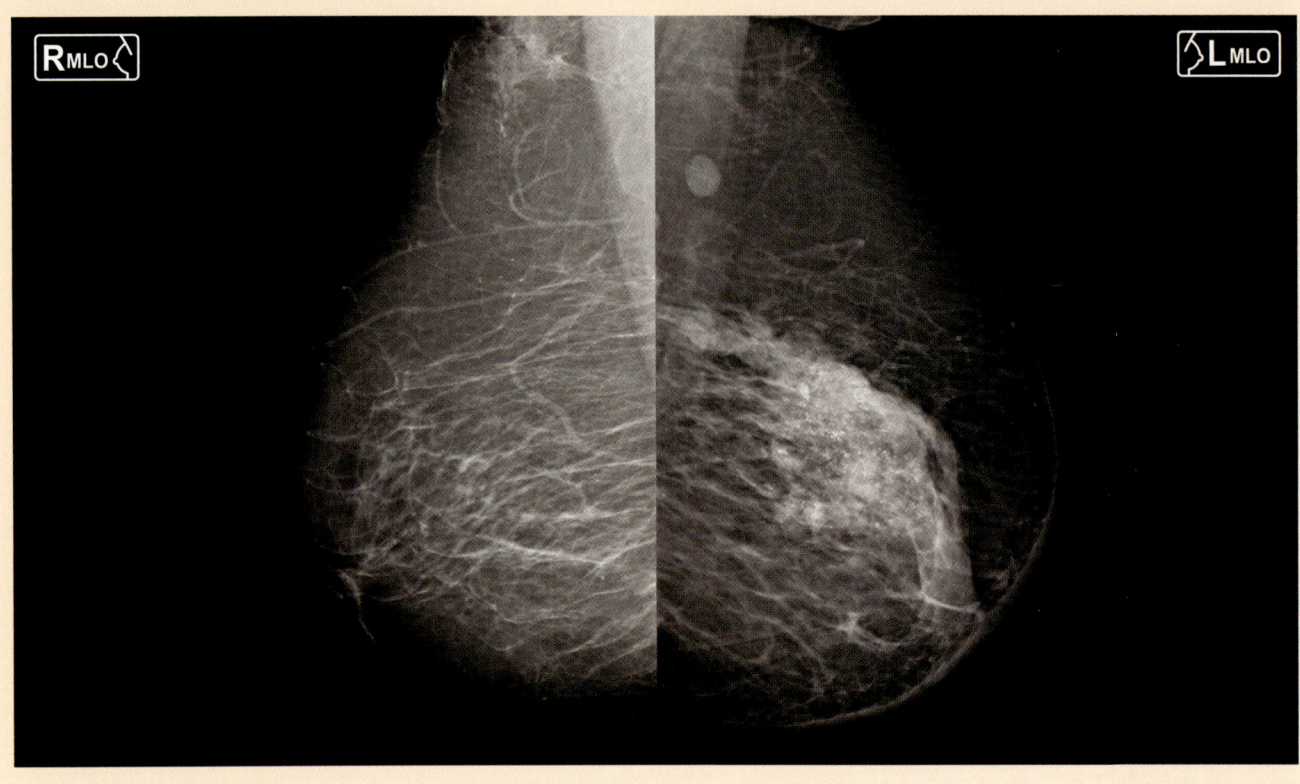

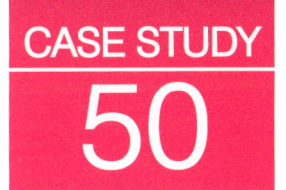
66-year-old lady, post-MRM for Ca left breast, for screening of right breast

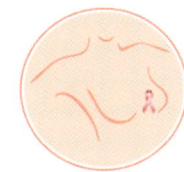

ACR Type B density.

Tiny punctate calcifications seen scattered in breast with mild clustering in upper-outer quadrant. BIRADS II/IV, suggested short-term follow-up/stereotactic biopsy. Follow-up mammography showed a few new punctate calcifications in the cluster of punctate calcifications in upper-outer quadrant. BIRADS IV, suggested stereotactic biopsy.

Stereotactic biopsy HPE: DCIS with no invasive component.

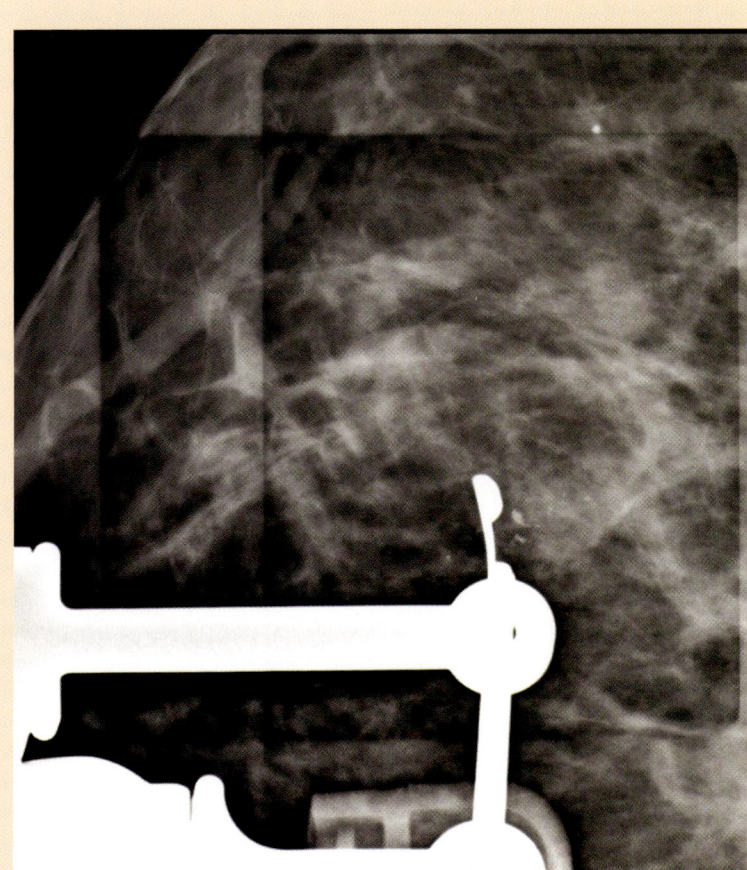

Sterotactic Biopsy

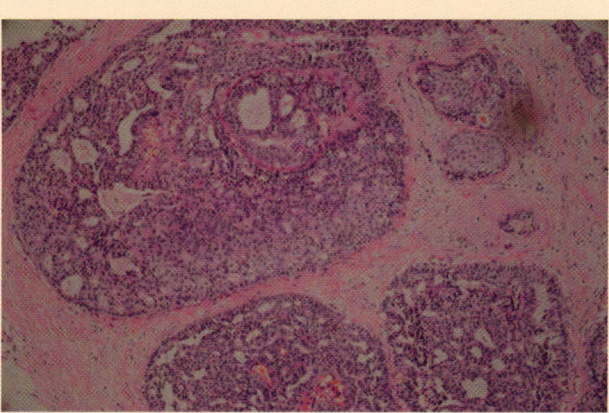

HPE image

Key Points

Any increase in size/added new punctate calcifications in a cluster of punctate calcifications should be viewed with suspicion and subjected to stereotactic biopsy as in this case.

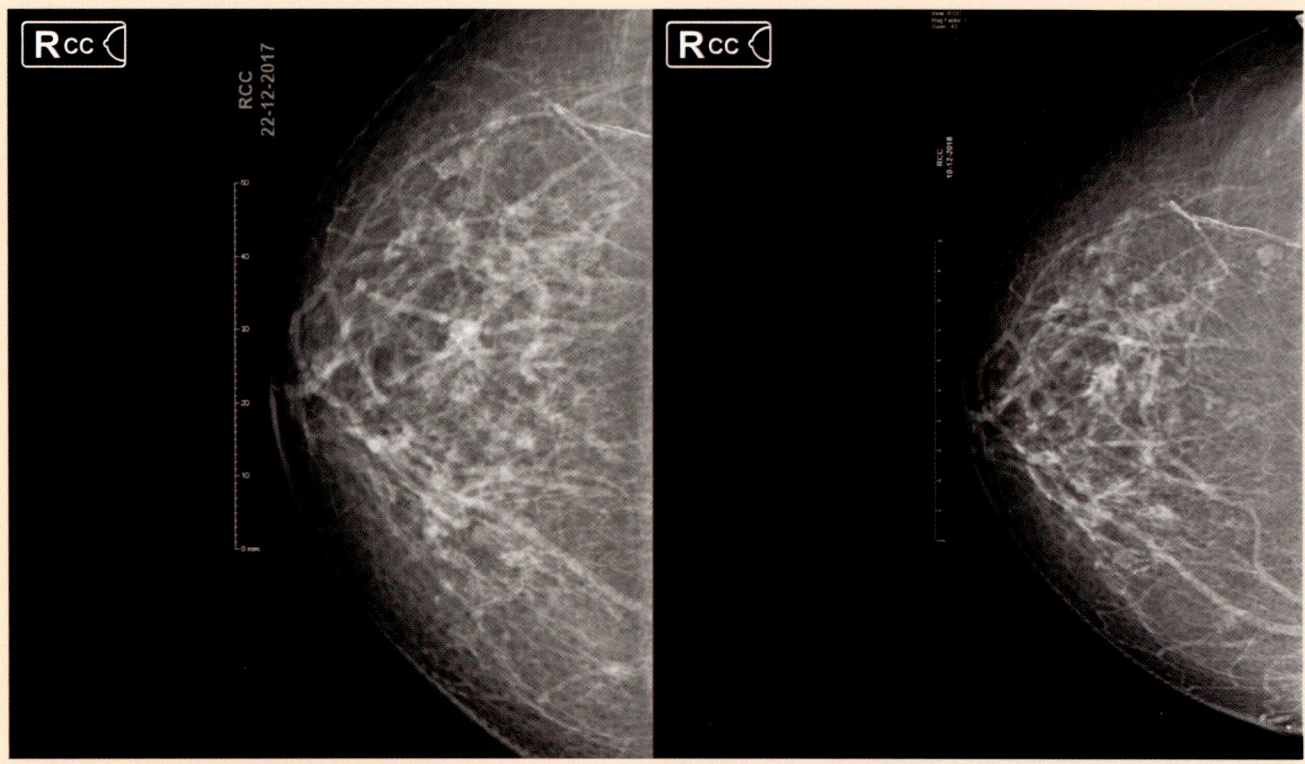

Right CC View Prior   Right CC View Current

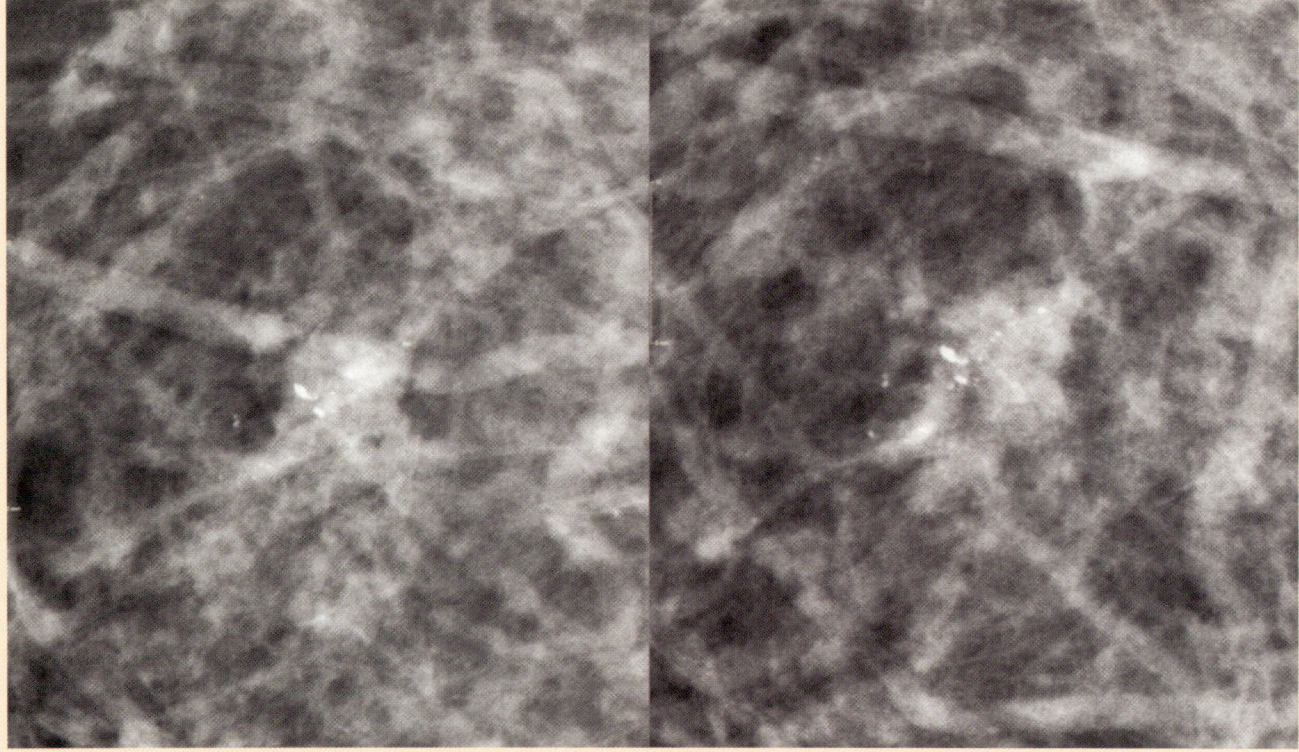

Zoomed Right CC Prior   Zoomed Right CC Current

Conclusion

FFDM is a reliable screening and diagnostic modality for picking up sub-clinical breast cancers and characterizing clinically palpable breast abnormalities. Stereotactic biopsy is a highly accurate method for HPE evaluation of tiny breast lesions, which may not be feasible to undergo guided biopsy by any other imaging modality. Combination of FFDM and stereotactic biopsy make a significant impact on bringing down breast cancer related mortality by helping in establishing pathological diagnosis of breast cancer in its early stage.